THE ENGINE 2 DIET

Books by Rip Esselstyn

The Engine 2 Diet

Plant-Strong

The Engine 2 Seven-Day Rescue Diet

The Engine 2 Cookbook

The

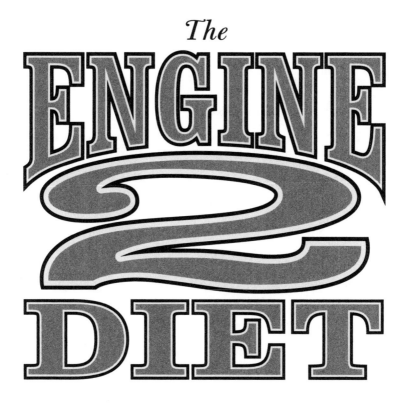

ENGINE 2 DIET

The Texas Firefighter's
28-Day Save-Your-Life Plan
That Lowers Cholesterol and
Burns Away the Pounds

RIP ESSELSTYN

GRAND CENTRAL
Life 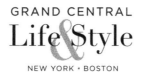 Style
NEW YORK · BOSTON

Grand Central Life & Style
Hachette Book Group
1290 Avenue of the Americas, New York, NY 10104
grandcentrallifeandstyle.com
twitter.com/grandcentralpub

First hardcover edition published by Wellness Central in 2009
First Grand Central Life & Style Trade Edition: December 2017

Grand Central Life & Style is an imprint of Grand Central Publishing. The Grand Central Life & Style name and logo are trademarks of Hachette Book Group, Inc.

The publisher is not responsible for websites (or their content) that are not owned by the publisher.

The Hachette Speakers Bureau provides a wide range of authors for speaking events. To find out more, go to www.hachettespeakersbureau.com or call (866) 376-6591.

"E2-Approved Foods to Keep in Your Pantry" on page 127 are copyright © 2016 by Rip Esselstyn and are reprinted from *The Engine 2 Seven-Day Rescue Diet.*

Print book interior design by HRoberts Design

Library of Congress Cataloging-in-Publication Data

Esselstyn, Rip.
   The Engine 2 diet: The Texas firefighter's 28-day save-your-life plan that lowers cholesterol and burns away the pounds / Rip Esselstyn.—1st ed.
      p. cm.
Includes index
   ISBN 978-0-446-50669-4
1. Reducing diets. 2. Vegetarianism. 3. Fire fighters—Texas. I. Title.
RM222.2 .E86 2009
613.2/5—dc22
                          2008046709

ISBNs: 978-0-446-50669-4 (hardcover); 978-0-446-50668-7 (trade paperback); 978-0-446-54368-2 (e-book)

Printed in the United States of America

LSC-C

10   9   8   7   6   5   4   3   2

For my wife, Jill, and my children Kole, Sophie, and Hope

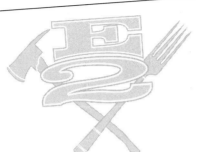

Dear Reader:

I'm Rip Esselstyn and I want to thank you for picking up my book. I hope that once you've read it, you will choose to embark on the Engine 2 Diet in what will be a spectacular health makeover. Think about it: In just twenty-eight days, you will plant the seeds of a long-lasting, healthy life. I know that if I didn't follow this diet, I would never have had the energy to be a world-class triathlete, or just as grueling, a firefighter.

The Engine 2 Diet is a snap to follow. Depending on which of two programs you select, you will spend either two or four weeks eating nothing but the most colorful, nutrient-packed foods Mother Nature provides: fruits, vegetables, whole grains, legumes, nuts, and seeds. During this time period you will push to the back burner all meats and dairy products, as well as refined and processed foods—including extracted oils—while feasting on jillions of plant-diverse foods.

That's the Engine 2 Diet in a healthy nutshell!

To assist you on your quest for great health, I have also included more than one hundred recipes that will make your mouth water, your friends envious, and your body happy.

I wish you only the best as you start what I hope will be a lifelong love affair with plant-beautiful foods. Remember, this isn't just a diet, it's an adventure in perfect health.

Eat Plant-Strong!

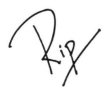

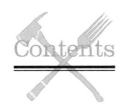

Contents

Foreword by T. Colin Campbell / xi

I. **The E2 Diet** / 1

1. Engine 2 / 3
2. My Story / 9
3. The Engine 2 Diet / 15
4. Crazy Myths About Food / 31
5. The Medical Proof Behind the Engine 2 Diet / 41
6. The E2 Exercise Program / 69

II. **Making It Work** / 87

1. The E2 Attitude / 89
2. E2 Vital Signs / 97
3. Label Reading / 107
4. Making It Work for Life! / 119

III. **Recipes and Meal Plans** / 121

Introduction / 123

1. Getting Your Kitchen in E2 Shape / 127
2. E2 Easy Weekly Planner / 143
3. E2 Recipes / 147

Acknowledgments / 257

Index / 261

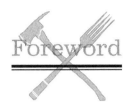

Foreword

The evidence is now in. What our grandmothers always told us to do—eat your vegetables and have an apple a day to keep the doctor away—is borne out by modern science. Increasingly, medical research is showing that we should consume a plant-based diet for optimal health.

But do people take this message seriously? I wish they did, but most do not. Part of the reason is our cultural tradition. For too long we have been accustomed, taste-wise, to animal foods or foods and food supplements derived from the wrong parts of plants, like their sugars, their oils (some of which we solidify and convert to trans fats!), and their refined flours without their outer bran layers. Then we add salt to produce unhealthy products that find their way to store shelves as convenience foods.

As a result, we've been getting fatter and suffering from an ever-increasing number and variety of ailments and life-threatening diseases. America now has the highest per capita health care costs in the world, while ignoring its many millions of citizens who lack medical insurance. Consuming the right kind of plant-based foods can go a long way toward solving not only our own personal health concerns, but our society's ills as well. There is simply nothing that can so profoundly affect our healing as eating fruits and vegetables.

How can we drive this message home? That is where Rip Esselstyn comes in. What a story he has to tell! It's personal, it's inspiring, and it's lifesaving. A world-class athlete and a firefighter, Rip managed to convert a firehouse full of committed meat eaters to a plant-based diet, and in the process improved everything from their weight to their blood pressure and cholesterol. From there he branched out to a pilot group of sixty-five volunteers, all of whom achieved the same stunning results as the firefighters—an average weight loss of ten pounds and a dramatic decline in cholesterol—in a mere four weeks.

Best of all, those who completed the program reported feeling so much better—with improvements to conditions such as kidney stones, constipation, and low energy—that few felt tempted to resume their old way of eating.

I am not surprised by Rip's accomplishments and motivations. He comes from an extraordinary line of medical men and women. The Esselstyns and the Criles (his mother's side) have served the public good for generations, and they know as much about medicine as any family in America. I find it fascinating that Rip, representing the first generation of the merger of these two brilliant medical families, has chosen to share his experiences in what I believe to be the most important health message to come upon the public horizon in many years.

I first met Rip in 1991 at a medical conference organized and hosted by his famous father, Dr. Caldwell B. Esselstyn, Jr., who was sharing for the first time his dramatic results on reversing and curing heart disease. He boldly named the conference "The First National Conference on the Elimination of Coronary Heart Disease" and had invited other researchers to present our own findings. Rip was only able to attend part of the conference, because of a prior commitment to compete in the Escape from Alcatraz Triathlon, but he had stopped by to get a sense of what his father and others were doing. I met Rip on three other occasions while I was lecturing in Austin, Texas. On one of those occasions, he introduced me to his Engine 2 firehouse buddies, and I sensed a remarkable story emerging that is now being told in these pages.

I have spent five decades working as an experimental research scientist in the field of diet and health. I believe in the message that Rip Esslestyn is advocating and that his father and other clinicians have been adopting with great success in their clinics. I was not drawn to this view by any particular ideology but because of the experimental research done in my laboratory (mostly at Cornell University). Our findings were often challenging, even difficult to accept at times, because my background, both personally and professionally, ran counter to what I was seeing. I was raised on a dairy farm, milking cows, and my family lived off the land.

As our evidence accumulated, it became ever more impressive. John McDougall, MD, for years has been treating people, with great success, for a variety of illnesses with the plant-based diet that Rip recommends in this book. Recently, he and other physicians have cured most of the Type

2 diabetics in their practices and, in many cases, have greatly reduced insulin needs even for Type 1 patients. Rip's father, Caldwell B. Esselstyn, Jr., MD, reverses and even cures advanced heart disease with this diet. Roy Swank, MD, followed multiple sclerosis patients for thirty-four years, using very much this same type of diet, and concluded that "about 95 percent of MS patients [diagnosed early] remained only mildly disabled for approximately thirty years."

I have been lecturing extensively around the country and have heard from many cancer patients that they believe that they are cured or at least are in remission because of using a plant-based diet. This belief is borne out by the findings in our extensive experimental animal studies, in which we could turn on and off cancer development by relatively modest nutritional means, using a model of this same diet. Obesity can be controlled, migraine headaches reduced, arthritic conditions alleviated—the list goes on and on. The idea that Rip Esselstyn elaborates in this book is "spot-on," as my associates across the big pond say.

I predict that this book will be as effective as any on the market in conveying an exceptionally important health message in a most personal way. Just read it, and you will see what I mean.

T. Colin Campbell, PhD
Professor Emeritus of Nutritional Biochemistry
Cornell University, Ithaca, New York

Co-author (with Thomas M. Campbell II) of
The China Study (2005)

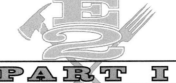

PART I

The
E2
Diet

1

ENGINE 2

The evening of January 5, 2000, was bitterly cold, a night no one in the Austin, Texas, fire department will soon forget. At the time I was working at Central Station, the city's largest. Central was called "The Animal House" because we firefighters were notorious for our bizarre antics, from launching water balloons at passersby from the second-story rooftop to breaking rookies down until they burst into tears. There were no barriers and no boundaries.

The weather was bad when we went to bed in the firehouse dorm that night, but by early morning it was worse: A freezing rain was falling, and temperatures were heading toward record lows. Then, at 4:20 a.m., a heavy box alarm sounded. (The word "box" refers to a home; a regular box alarm signals that a single-family house is on fire, but when a heavy box alarm sounds, it means a fire at a larger building, such as an apartment complex.)

Just as at the start of an athletic competition, all my senses went into overdrive—my heart rate jumped, my stomach churned, my mind raced. Normally I'd leap right out of bed, jump into my bunker pants, and pull up my suspenders, but because I was going to be driving this shift, I had only enough time to stumble into my station pants and cotton shirt before sliding down the eighteen-foot brass fire pole.

I was also preparing for the worst. The real burners generally occur between midnight and 6:00 a.m., when people have gone to sleep but a stovetop is left burning, an electrical wire shorts out, or a smoldering cigarette butt ignites.

The fire turned out to be at the Lake Shore Apartments, two-and-a-half miles from the station. Sirens blaring, we pulled up to the scene, the third engine in. (Each arriving engine has a specific duty. The first engine attacks the fire, the second backs up the first, and the third hooks up to a hydrant to bring an unlimited supply of water to the first.)

Just as we were arriving, we heard a radio message from Engine 22, announcing that they had put out the fire. For a moment we relaxed, and from where we stood, looking up at the building's second-floor balcony, the problem seemed to be nothing more than a little hibachi fire.

Then my good friend, fellow Engine 1 firefighter Josh Miller, said, "Rip, put your bunker gear on." I didn't understand why he'd told me that, because things seemed to be under control. Perhaps he'd had a premonition—all firefighters have them—so I listened, scuttled around to the driver's side compartment, and donned my full gear.

Sure enough, moments later that little fire exploded into enormous flames—larger than I had ever seen. They climbed up the side of the building, curled onto its top, and engulfed the roof.

Scared and nervous, I approached the fire, my pulse pounding. The next few minutes were a blur; time warps under severe pressure. I remember that a firefighter named Alphonse Dellert, known as Ax, stepped in front of me, and as he did, I heard the kind of bloodcurdling screams you hear only in movies: "Help me, I'm burning up!" I wasn't sure I'd heard correctly, but then the cry came again: "Help me, I'm burning!"

I sensed this scream was coming from the apartment with the balcony—but how could someone still be alive inside that inferno? The flames were rising even higher and their radiant heat was overwhelming, even from two hundred feet away.

Ax and I were the only ones who heard the screams. Ax sprang into action. He put on his face piece, went on air (we all carry bottles supplying forty-five minutes of air so we can breathe during the worst fires), grabbed a rack line (a preconnected two-hundred-foot hose), and scrambled up a ladder. Right behind Ax, I also went on air, then steadied the ladder for him, although he was too preoccupied to realize I was watching his every move.

Ax reached the window's edge, opened the hose, and sprayed torrents of water into the left side of the apartment, the heart of the flames. Then he hung the hose's nozzle on the ladder's top rung and entered the window, disappearing into the inferno.

All I could think was: I have to protect him. So I climbed the ladder and looked in the window. It felt as if I were peering at a secret passage into Hell.

A friend of mine once served as the medical director at Yosemite National Park, where, several years ago, a lunatic had beheaded one woman and killed three others. My friend went out to locate the victims, but all he found was one headless body. At that point his reality changed; he'd come to believe in true evil. That's how I felt then, seeing the fiery monster raging, laughing at us: "I'm loving this, and you guys are screwed."

Because it was difficult to see, I had no idea who was trapped inside the apartment. Later we discovered it was Fire Captain John Butz. John belonged to the first-arriving ladder company, which was responsible for search and rescue. John had entered the apartment with his crew, but as they had forgotten to bring a fan along to ventilate the room, he'd sent them back to get it and had gone in alone—even though we're always supposed to bring a partner and a charged hose line (one that holds water at the appropriate pressure).

Before John had had time to exit the room he was investigating, the living room next door flashed (anything reaching 1,000 degrees or higher will burst into flames). If John had been inside, he would have died on the spot. Instead, the explosion threw him to the ground, where he lay paralyzed and could only scream for help. The flames and smoke were so dense that Ax couldn't find John until he spotted his flashlight at the end of the bed. Ax knelt down and asked, "Can you make it to the window?" John whispered, "I'll do what I can."

Ax turned around, trying to orient himself amid the smoke and flames. At that moment I entered through the window, waving my arms—Ax saw my silhouette and headed for it. Later he called me his angel.

The distance from the floor to the bottom edge of the window was four feet, so the two of us began struggling to raise John's limp 300 pounds up and over the sill. (John weighed about 225 pounds, but was also wearing 75 pounds of equipment.)

Meanwhile, the freezing rain was still falling, and the smoke was impairing our vision. I slipped on the ladder, John's helmet fell off, and we still couldn't pull his limp body past the windowsill.

Finally, we got the front half of his body to dangle over the sill. Ax yelled, "Do you have him?"

"I got him," I yelled back, yanking John as best I could out and over the window so I could lower him. At this point I wasn't sure if he was still alive. I bear-hugged the ladder with my left arm, lowering John until my right arm was fully extended, and then let him fall. He dropped eighteen feet to the ground, missing an enormous air-conditioning unit by inches.

Next, I climbed back up the ladder looking for Ax, who, in the confusion, I mistook for my friend Josh Miller—at this point I was so befuddled I didn't know who was who. But I was not going anywhere without the other firefighter, and because I was convinced he was inside, I was about to reenter the room. Then something inside me said, "Look down and see what's on the ground."

I did, and lying eighteen feet below were both John Butz and Ax. Their bodies were smoking.

At this point I had no idea how Ax had landed there. I later learned that he was so hot, and suffering from such severe injuries, that to save his own life he had dived over the ladder and fallen to the ground. I had been so busy wrestling with John's body that I didn't see him.

I made my way down the ladder to Ax and John. Incredibly, both were still conscious. Ax had third-degree burns to his calf, hands, and neck. John was not as lucky; third-degree burns covered close to 70 percent of his body. People seldom live if more than 65 percent of the body is burned.

Finally, the fire was contained. John was taken by ambulance to Brackenridge Hospital, then airlifted to Brooke Army Medical Center in San Antonio, where he spent almost a year in recovery. Shortly afterward, he was promoted from captain to battalion chief. He is lucky to be alive, and he knows it.

Although two later sweeps of the apartment revealed no other victims, the third sweep found a man dead in the bathtub. The shower curtain had melted over his body, which was barely recognizable as human. The apartment had been his, and his little hibachi had caused the deadly blaze.

That fire's fury spooked me to the core. In the short time all these events took place, I realized how fleeting our time on earth is. Since that night, I've appreciated the importance of my job, as well as the other firefighters with whom I work, more than ever before. I never take a single shift for granted—and after twenty-four hours, when we're relieved by the next crew, I heave a sigh of relief knowing that we'll all go home safely.

That terrible fire also confirmed my belief that we can't take anything for granted—especially our health. Obviously, preventing and staying away from fire is one way to stay healthy. But the most basic, profound, and powerful way to take care of your health on a day-to-day basis is to eat a healthy, plant-based diet. This regimen is the best way to fight the dangerous fires raging inside us—fires that create all the chronic Western ailments including heart attack, stroke, cancer, Alzheimer's disease, and diabetes. That's why I created the Engine 2 Diet, and why I wrote this book.

2

MY STORY

ll my life I've been intrigued by health, performance, and diet. As long as I can remember a chin-up bar hung on the door of my bedroom, where I worked out religiously several times a day. In the sixth grade, I set the school record with twenty-two. At the age of twelve, after watching the movie *Rocky*, I immediately came home and downed a glass filled with raw eggs. At thirteen, my father bought free weights, dumbbells, and a Universal weight-lifting machine for the family playroom. They were well worn within a few years.

While I was in school, athletics were my stage. I set many high school swimming records (and still hold a national record in the 200-meter medley relay); I was the top player on my high school tennis team and co-captain of the water polo team.

As a young athlete, I lived on bacon, steaks, and triple cheeseburgers, thinking that such a diet was good for me and my performance. But that all changed in 1986, once I graduated from the University of Texas at Austin (where I was a three-time All-American swimmer and an Olympic trials qualifier in the 100- and 200-meter backstroke and freestyle events). Within six months I was competing as a professional triathlete and fueling my body with healthy foods that were a far cry from what I had known.

This shift was inspired by my father's groundbreaking research on plant-based diets, about which you will soon be reading, as well as by many great athletes who relied on a vegetarian diet for optimum performance, including six-time Hawaii Ironman champion Dave Scott, famed 400-meter hurdler Edwin Moses, and tennis great Martina Navratilova.

As a professional triathlete, I competed around the world in the Olympic distance triathlon (a 1-mile swim, 24.8-mile bike ride, and 6.2-mile run), and for many years was ranked as one of the country's top ten triathletes—and for most of that time, the sport's preeminent swimmer. Throughout this period I maintained a plant-strong diet in order to enhance my recovery between two and three daily workouts, and to give me an edge on race day.

The diet worked: I took first place in many major events, including the world's largest athletic competition, the World Police and Fire Games, in 2001. I've also won the Capital of Texas Triathlon eight times, and have been the leader or top-three finisher at many televised events, including the Escape from Alcatraz Triathlon, where I was first out of the frigid, shark-infested waters six years in a row.

In 1997, knowing I couldn't be a professional athlete forever, I looked around for something new, and when several triathlete/firefighter friends suggested I consider firefighting, I listened. They described the job as twenty-four hours of adrenaline-pumping excitement, with no two shifts ever the same—a career in which you never had to sit behind a desk or take paperwork home on weekends. And there was the chance to help people as well. It was an easy decision.

Fighting fires and racing triathlons are animals of a different color: Training for and competing in triathlons is predictable; firefighting is not. There is no telling when the next alarm will sound and what the nature of the call will be, from a fire in a Dumpster or a high-rise to a medical call or an accident. The best way to stay on top of your game is to consistently fuel your body with clean-burning, artery-scrubbing, disease-reversing, and energy-giving plant-powered foods.

And so I always do, and still manage to compete as a world-class triathlete as well—in 2005, I participated in the Xterra World Championship on the Hawaiian island of Maui; the next year, at the age of forty-three, I was named one of Austin's ten fittest people. In May 2008, I set the national record at the U.S. Masters Swimming championships in the 200-yard backstroke.

My commitment to a healthy plant-based life has resulted in many people asking me to help them with their diets. So in 2006, I devised a six-week study and put fifty-eight people through a gauntlet of before-and-after tests to quantify the results, which were spectacular!

Then, in 2008, I initiated a four-week study and got more great results. It's one thing to say the diet works; it's another when you have tangible data that confirms the benefits of a plant-based diet. (You can read more about these studies in The Medical Proof Behind the Engine 2 Diet, page 41.)

One of the reasons I came up with these tests is that I come from a long line of trailblazing physicians. In fact, I was bred to be healthy—there aren't many families in America more dedicated to well-being than mine.

My father, Caldwell B. Esselstyn, Jr., MD, has always been my hero. He was also the son of a great doctor, Caldwell B. Esselstyn, Sr., who was baseball star Lou Gehrig's personal physician as well as founder of the Rip Van Winkle Clinic in upstate New York, where people such as Eleanor Roosevelt sought medical help.

After graduating from Yale and winning a gold medal in rowing at the 1956 Summer Olympic Games, my father attended Case Western Reserve Medical School, then did his internship and residency at the Cleveland Clinic. One of the world's finest medical facilities, the clinic was founded by my mother's great-grandfather, George Crile, Sr. During my father's tenure there, he was honored with numerous awards and held many offices, including president of the clinic's medical staff, member of its Board of Governors, and chairman of its Breast Cancer Task Force.

Most relevant to this book was the study my father initiated on the arrest and reversal of heart disease through diet—research that is still ongoing nearly thirty years later.

Frustrated with surgery as a means of treating disease, my father became convinced there was a better way to address the problem rather than simply treating its symptoms. By examining data from other cultures and countries, he had come to realize that diet must play a crucial role in human health—although at that time few doctors believed that health and nutrition were closely related.

My father's study began after he asked the Cleveland Clinic's cardiology department to send him patients afflicted with serious heart disease—people who had failed their bypass operations or their angioplasties, or who were too sick for these procedures, or who had refused these interventions entirely. He ended up working with eighteen people who had suffered forty-nine coronary events over the previous eight years.

Theorizing that a healthier diet would improve the patients' heart health, my father put them on a plant-based eating plan similar to the Engine 2 Diet. He eventually published the results in more than seven peer-reviewed medical journals including *The American Journal of Cardiology*, later updating his findings for his book *Prevent and Reverse Heart Disease* (Avery, 2007).

(The patients were also given very low doses of a cholesterol-lowering statin because, as my father said, he wanted to make sure they "were not only wearing a belt but also suspenders.")

These findings showed that of the patients reviewed after a dozen years, all but one suffered no further coronary events—and that single patient who did had strayed from my father's diet.

Moreover, these people stopped the disease dead in its tracks, and all of them lived long lives. (Those who have since died succumbed to non-heart-related conditions.)

Furthermore, every single participant's health markers improved as well. Their overall cholesterol level dropped below 150 mg/dl, a magic number as studies have repeatedly shown that heart disease is exceedingly rare among people with total cholesterol levels under 150.

Note: Cholesterol is measured in milligrams per deciliter, which is abbreviated "mg/dl." For ease of reading I have taken out the unit of measurement "mg/dl" after many of the cholesterol levels.

One of the most intriguing cases from my father's study is that of Dr. Joseph Crow, a fellow general surgeon who had taken over my father's position as chairman of the Cleveland Clinic's Breast Cancer Task Force. One day, forty-four-year-old Joe had just finished operating when he suffered a full-blown heart attack. Joe didn't smoke and wasn't overweight, had no prior history—nor family history—of heart disease, and his total cholesterol was a respectable 156. But his heart was a mess.

Owing to the nature of Joe's arterial blockage, he was not a candidate for surgery or stents, and he refused to take cholesterol-lowering drugs. So he knocked on my father's office door, and soon became a faithful plant-based eater.

Over the span of the next two-and-a-half years, Joe completely reversed the blockages in the portion of his heart known as the left anterior descending coronary artery. He also brought his total cholesterol down from 156 to 89, and reduced his lethal LDL cholesterol from 98 to 38. All of this with one course of treatment—a hard-core, plant-strong diet!

Now that my father had become convinced that so many people were becoming sick because of their diet, he decided that if he was going to make his patients eat a certain way, his family was going to do so, too. We had always eaten the usual American diet of roast beef, cheese, and eggs, but soon enough, our whole family was eating a healthy, plant-based diet.

My mother jumped on board because she was not only the wife of a great doctor but also the daughter of one—George "Barney" Crile, one of the most influential physicians of his generation. After graduating summa cum laude from Harvard Medical School in 1933, Barney eventually went to work at the Cleveland Clinic.

Often called "The Savior of the American Breast," Barney was the first American surgeon to perform the breast-conserving partial mastectomy operation, rather than the routine practice of the total mastectomy, on women with breast cancer.

E2 POP QUIZ

Q: What are the magic numbers you want your total and LDL cholesterol levels to be so your body starts clearing away existing plaque formations?

A: You want a total cholesterol level below 150 and an LDL cholesterol level below 80.

Barney's father, George Crile, Sr., who, as mentioned, founded the Cleveland Clinic, was considered one of the great surgeons of the twentieth century. He was responsible for many firsts, including the first human-to-human blood transfusion, and was a co-founder of the American Red Cross. He and Barney are the only American father and son ever to be inducted into England's Royal College of Surgeons.

*   *   *

IT'S NOW 2018, AND I'M NO LONGER FIGHTING fires with the Austin Fire Department, but I'm fighting chronic Western diseases together with Whole Foods Market. I spend my days teaching people how to transform their health by eating a whole food, plant-based (plant-strong) diet. The firefighter in me will always want to help people and save lives—I believe that dragging you away from your disease-promoting diet and toward a better way of life will have just as profound an impact as dragging you out of a raging fire.

3

THE ENGINE 2 DIET

HOW IT ALL BEGAN

There's no argument that the Engine 2 Diet can protect you from disease while making you feel and look terrific. But the diet might actually never have been created if it weren't for an argument.

Although we are often harried, there is still occasional downtime between calls at the firehouse known as Engine 2, which is nestled on the outskirts of the University of Texas campus (I transferred here from downtown Austin's Central Station in January 2002). So we're constantly coming up with ways to keep ourselves busy. The competitions are endless: Who can climb the fire pole hand over hand without using his feet? Who rules the roost when it comes to Ping-Pong? Who can collect the most money in his firefighter boot for Jerry's Kids, our annual muscular dystrophy fund-raiser? Who can hoist the 180-pound dummy over his shoulder, carry it up the back stairs, through the dormitory, and down the front stairs in the shortest amount of time?

So one day in 2003, when James Rae (aka JR), Josh Miller, and I were sitting on the station's front porch, we started talking about health and cholesterol levels, and as always, the discussion soon became a squabble over whose cholesterol level was lowest. I was sure mine was, but so was Josh. JR, who had no idea, wanted to play along, so the next morning the three of us drove over to the People's Rx and had our cholesterol levels checked. Josh's level turned out to be 168, mine was 199, but JR's was a whopping 344.

My level, much higher than I had expected, caused me to lose the bet. But I had an excuse: The day before, I had raced in the Dirty Duathlon (a 5-kilometer trail run, followed by a 25-kilometer mountain bike ride, ending with another 5-kilometer trail run), competing against my ex-triathlon competitor and friend Lance Armstrong and a slew of others (I came in third, Lance was first). As a reward, I let myself eat my once-a-year cheeseburger with all the trimmings—not something you want to do just before a cholesterol test and not something I've ever done again.

But because JR's cholesterol was so high, it took all the heat off me.

It turned out that all the males in the Rae family had died of heart disease before the age of fifty-two, except JR's father, who had undergone triple bypass surgery at fifty-four. As one of the fire department lieutenants said when he heard about JR's tests: "The man's a walking heart attack." Furthermore, JR was married, the father of two young children, and only thirty-three years old.

So rather than pulling JR out of a fire someday, we decided to rescue him through a healthy diet.

I had always eaten well at the station. Sometimes JR and Josh would join me in dining on my plant-based creations. But now we made a concerted effort to start a healthy lunch wagon. (A wagon is a family-style meal in which we help each other prep, cook, and then clean up; it's a cultural tradition at firehouses throughout the world.) Every day we prepared wholesome sandwiches, tacos, veggie burgers, and wraps with hummus and vegetables on whole wheat or corn tortillas.

A few months later, when the Austin Fire Department held a contest for the healthiest lunch wagon, Engine 2 entered and won—another notch in our competitive belts.

Over the next year and a half, given our tendency to do everything to its fullest extent, and to support JR on his quest to buck the Rae family tradition, we developed a full-blown, plant-based eating schedule around our twenty-four-hour shift: lunch when we arrived at noon, dinner that evening, breakfast the next morning, and lunch before we left for home again at noon.

A year later, JR had his cholesterol checked again. It had only come down to the 270s. I suspected he needed to commit to our eating lifestyle at home as well as at the firehouse, so I asked JR to eat all plant-based for just three weeks, then have his cholesterol level checked once more.

The results? His cholesterol had plummeted to an impressive 196—a drop of 146 points (or 57 percent) from his high of 344!

E2 POP QUIZ

Q: What percentage of heart attacks occur with people who have supposedly heart-healthy cholesterol levels?

A: Thirty-five percent of all heart attacks occur in people with a total cholesterol between 150 and 199 mg/dl, numbers most physicians and the American Heart Association consider desirable.

THE ENGINE 2 PILOT STUDY

Truly my father's son, I decided at this point that it was necessary to complete a more formal study to prove the effectiveness of the Engine 2 Diet. I wanted to bring more people on board to show the dramatic impact of an all-out, plant-based diet on a wide cross-section of people, from professional athletes to working moms and dads, from couples to singles, from meat eaters to vegetarians, from the very healthy to the not-so-healthy.

By the winter of 2006, armed with a medical director (a doctor for the Travis County Sheriff's Office), a community website, and a lab to test lipid profiles, I was ready. Now all I needed were participants to make the Engine 2 Pilot Study a reality.

I put out the word, hoping to find two dozen volunteers. Within two weeks, I had to cap the number at sixty-five. Far more people than I'd expected were ready and willing to clean up their diets and their lives.

Among my volunteers were my thirteen-year-old next-door neighbor, grandparents, vegans, cancer survivors, world-class triathletes, multiple sclerosis patients, lawyers, business owners, and doctors. Also included were a few additional firefighters (male and female), a storm chaser, and the director of advancement for the Lance Armstrong Foundation.

Several people had to drop out, and some people joined in a few days late, but all in all, fifty-eight people finished the six-week program.

And they got results! The study was a raging success.

The level of that success can be measured by the before-and-after markers I used to track changes in participants' health. Before starting the diet, everyone in the study took medical tests to obtain benchmarks for everything from weight and blood pressure to a full lipid profile, which includes total cholesterol level, LDL cholesterol, HDL cholesterol, risk ratio (LDL/HDL), and triglycerides.

After finishing the program, these markers were checked again.

(In Engine 2 Vital Signs, page 97, I will explain in more detail what these markers mean, and ask you to have them checked so you can track your own magnificent success. But for those of you who have trouble remembering: LDL is your bad, or lethal, cholesterol, and HDL is your good, or healthy, cholesterol.)

The most impressive result was the decrease in the group's average overall cholesterol level from 181 mg/dl to 142 mg/dl, an average drop of 39 points, bringing them well below the magic number of 150, which makes you heart attack proof.

The average LDL cholesterol fell from 109 to 77, a drop of 32 points, also bringing them below the second magic number, 80, which not only makes you heart attack proof, but also helps you to become resistant to other chronic diseases.

The greatest total cholesterol drop for an individual was 91 points (from 216 to 125), and the greatest LDL drop, 78 points (from 189 to 111). We also saw a total mean weight loss of 10 pounds, and our group average weight fell from 172 to 162 pounds. The average weight loss for men was 15.0 pounds, and for women, 8.5 pounds.

The significant weight loss was particularly startling because not everyone in the Pilot Study had wanted to lose weight—many became involved solely for the health benefits. Still, the women lost between 2 and 26 pounds, and the men lost between 2 and 31 pounds.

Furthermore, the participants noted that other conditions—from kidney stones to acne, from constipation to low energy—also began clearing up.

Here are some of their stories:

THE SECOND STUDY

On June 5, 2008, fifteen people (thirteen firefighters and two civilians) embarked on a second, twenty-eight-day Engine 2 Pilot Study. As with the first study, the results were mind-boggling! The group started with an average total cholesterol of 197 mg/dl. Twenty-eight days later, this number had dropped to 135, or 62 points (30 percent). The group started with an average LDL cholesterol of 124 mg/dl; this dropped to 74 mg/dl, or 50 points (40 percent). And the group's average weight went from 203 to 189 pounds, or an average loss of 14 pounds per person. This hard-core evidence shows the powerful results that are within the grasp of each and every one of you. This means you!

The ENGINE 2 DIET	Total Cholesterol Before	Total Cholesterol After	LDL Cholesterol Before	LDL Cholesterol After	Weight Before	Weight After
Jack Murray	243	150	168	91	177	167
Ramiro Zapata	232	142	150	77	201	185
Sean Cummings	227	144	151	89	161	149
John Wolfe	223	154	137	83	179	169
Don Barthlow	222	164	160	99	186	178
Josh Simpson	220	170	160	113	189	174
Lawrence Wesley	217	144	146	84	261	245
Mark Gruell	213	118	145	63	194	181
Gilbert Selvera	195	152	117	76	174	166
Drew Corbin	179	124	80	63	251	231
Tim Bosma	174	93	104	44	304	271
Seabrook Jones	174	136	117	69	199	184
Donnie Caldwell	156	123	93	73	208	196
Colin Camp	150	90	82	37	196	185
Louise Joubert	130	128	57	56	159	155
Group Averages: Group Average loss:	**197**	**135** −62 points	**124**	**74** −50 points	**203**	**189** −14 pounds

One man said that his sister, a vascular surgeon at a major Dallas hospital, found it hard to believe his total cholesterol level could drop from 214 to 135 in just a few weeks and wanted to make sure that he was firing on all cylinders. Because he'd had other health issues besides high cholesterol, she gave him a treadmill stress test to assess his overall fitness, which he aced. After that, and after reading several articles about my father's research on reversing heart disease, she asked her brother to send her photocopies of as many Engine 2 recipes as possible.

Another man, who lost 20 pounds and whose cholesterol dropped from 216 to 125, told me that he'd always imagined that little green men were working inside his body to repair all the damage he'd caused. But now that he'd been eating the Engine 2 way, he imagined them sitting around like the Maytag Repairman, bored and waiting for the phone to ring.

Several people talked about how their tastes had changed over the six weeks. "You don't need butter or cheese for food to taste good," one woman said, "and I never knew that before." Another woman said, "You actually taste the real food and not what it's covered with."

A physician participant said that he thought plant-based eating would be harsh on his taste buds, but after just a few weeks he noticed that his palate was changing: He no longer craved any of his old favorites, and found just the thought of eating meat, cheese, or eggs unpleasant.

A number of participants mentioned how they'd never realized what a wide array of food is available to plant eaters. They'd thought it was all about carrots and lettuce. Now they've learned that it's not called the plant *kingdom* for nothing.

Another subject that came up repeatedly was a change in bathroom habits. Every single participant said he or she was pooping at least twice a day—and sometimes up to four times—even though before the study many had only been going a few times a week. One of the women's doctors had told her that pooping twice a week was a normal condition called lazy bowel syndrome. But once on the Engine 2 Diet, within one week she started pooping once a day and twice a day thereafter.

Bowel movement improvement is one of the greatest rewards of a plant-based diet, so it became a hot topic of conversation. My own term for the act has always been "pooping," but my participants came up with some great phrases, such as "I now release hostages two to three times a day," "I drop the kids off at the pool more than ever," or from one of the triathletes: "I am spending far less time in the men's library."

The Pilot Study results were impressive, but the most important lesson I took from them was that it wasn't just firefighters who can profit from the E2 Diet. It's everyone and anyone who can fog a mirror or think a thought.

THE ENGINE 2 DIET

The Engine 2 Diet is a simple, easy-to-follow four-week program that will enable you to reach whatever goal you choose, whether it's losing weight, becoming physically fit, or reducing the precursors to disease, such as high cholesterol, high blood pressure, obesity, blockage of the arteries, high blood sugar, insulin resistance, or all of the above.

Colin J. Wallis, 37
Director of Advancement, Lance Armstrong Foundation

Think of it as a science project. Pay close attention to the inputs and outputs. Monitor your sleep, exercise, energy, strength, mood, and compare them with how you were on the traditional American diet. This creates a bit of a game, and makes it easy to have fun and see the results.

When you follow the Engine 2 Plan, you will:

- Lose weight
- Lose body fat
- Increase lean muscle mass
- Improve your cardiovascular health

- Free yourself from the shackles of chronic Western diseases
- Have fun learning how to make new, smart, and delicious food choices
- Improve self-esteem and confidence
- Be instilled with a sense of personal power, because you, and you alone, are in control of your health
- Absolutely love how you feel

The reason the program will help you lose weight is not because you will be painstakingly measuring your portions or warily watching your calories, but because you will be eating only satisfying, whole foods that are nutrient dense as well as naturally low in calories and high in fiber.

This kind of pure diet will also grant you clarity of mind and increased energy. Ask the firefighters at Engine 2: Derick Zwerneman said, "I feel clean and light." Josh Miller told me he felt as though his "whole system has been rebooted." And Steve Martinez commented, "My whole body and mind feel like your teeth do after a cleaning from the dental hygienist."

So let's begin!

THE TWO ENGINE 2 DIET PLANS

You have a choice of two plans—the *Fire Cadet* and the *Firefighter*.

For the most part, firefighters don't know how to do anything half-assed. So when I ask people to start the diet, I seldom seek moderation. I ask people to start at the highest possible level of commitment.

But for some, the diet can appear daunting, so I offer the Fire Cadet option for those who prefer a more gradual approach.

Others can charge right in with the Firefighter plan—which I recommend, because you'll be setting yourself on a course to achieve better results in terms of everything from weight loss to lowered cholesterol levels. And isn't that worth two extra weeks of work?

But if you do start with the Cadet plan, you can always change your mind and go full bore later. At the start of the E2 Pilot Study, the participants were divided almost evenly between the Firefighter and the Fire Cadet options. After the first week, however, almost 80 percent of the Fire Cadets called me to say they wanted to join the Firefighter plan.

Fire Cadet

The Fire Cadet option is for those who don't like rushing into things, yet still want to find that pot of health at the end of the rainbow. Over the first two weeks, the fire cadet will wean him- or herself off unfriendly foods while eating an abundance of healthy, delicious ones.

Week One: No dairy of any kind. This includes all dairy—milk, cheese, creams, yogurt, butter, ice cream, and sour cream.

Also, no processed or refined foods—and that means white rice, white flour, white pasta, white bread, and anything else that is processed: cakes, cookies, unhealthy chips, sodas, etc.

Week Two: Now you stop eating meat, chicken, eggs, and fish, and continue to avoid dairy and refined foods. In other words, no pork, no turkey, no buffalo, no venison. Nothing that paws a hoof or flaps a wing. Nothing with a face and nothing with a mother, on land or in water.

Week Three: Keep the lid on all oils. Yes, I want you to stop eating all added or extracted oils, whether they're olive, canola, coconut, or any other. We don't eat baked goods with added oils, we don't use salad dressings with added oils, and we don't cook with added oils.

Now you're doing the whole shebang: no dairy, no refined foods, no meat, and no oils.

Week Four: You're still on the total E2 diet. You are digging in with both heels and consuming only whole foods. You are living the dream! You are nourishing yourself with only the best and brightest foods on earth: fruits, vegetables, whole grains, legumes, nuts, and seeds.

Please check out Part III of this book to see some of the excellent meals you'll be enjoying—breakfasts, lunches, and dinners that include delicacies such as blueberry pancakes, French toast, pizzas, shepherd's pie, vegetable curries, mushroom burgers with sweet potato fries, orange mousse, and fruit pie.

Firefighter

Starting on Day One, the Firefighter will jump in with both feet, eating a diet filled with healthy whole grains, vegetables, fruits, and legumes, while abstaining from all animal-based products and refined foods. What the Fire Cadet will be practicing in Weeks Three and Four, the Firefighter will be practicing for all four weeks—and happily so!

THIS IS THE SIMPLEST PROGRAM you can imagine. And to make it even simpler, check out Part III's tips that make all this as easy as a healthy date nut crust pie. And speaking of pies, you'll also be able to eat delectable cookies, casseroles, breads, soups, and so much more. After a while, you won't even miss the foods you'll be avoiding—which we'll now talk about in a little more detail.

Week One—Dairy and Processed Foods

I think of dairy products as meat, only in a liquid, cream, or solid form. After all, they contain just as many concentrated, disease-promoting, and nutritionally compromised calories.

Dairy is ubiquitous in the American diet. The milk and dairy industries have done an amazing job of propagating and maintaining the myth that we need three servings of milk, cheese, and/or yogurt a day to maintain healthy bones and overall health. We don't. In fact, the opposite is true—see page 35.

So instead of reaching for a glass of milk, sample the many wonderful milk substitutes found in most supermarkets: soy, rice, almond, and oat milk, for example. Use any one of these in recipes calling for milk.

Also remember to avoid all cheeses. Cheese is, simply put, a disease-promoting, nutritionally vacant, calorie-dense food. It's loaded with saturated fat and animal protein. Cheese also contains casomorphines (i.e., low levels of morphine), which is why so many people have such a hard time kicking the cheese habit. No compromising here! No cheese for you!

And be wary of soy cheese substitutes, too, because they generally contain casein, which is not only the main protein found in dairy foods but also, according to many studies, is a major promoter of tumors and cancer.

Please pat the butter good-bye as well. Rather than disguising food with butter, why not appreciate vegetables and grains for their authentic and natural taste? Open up your spice cabinet, sprinkle some on, and discover an entirely new world of flavors. Use a nonstick spray (but only very little) to grease skillets, casseroles, baking sheets, and pans.

Think about it: when you eliminate all forms of dairy, you'll have neither allergens, nor lactose intolerance, nor animal protein, nor saturated fat to deal with, and a host of new foods and flavors to enjoy. It's a win-win choice.

Americans currently consume a staggering 50 percent of their calories from refined and processed foods. With no fiber and scant amounts of vitamins and minerals, these empty calories will be replaced immediately by whole foods. Whole foods are stocked with fiber, vitamins and minerals, and calories that count. Without cakes, cookies, soda pop, unhealthy chips, white rice, white flour, white pasta, and white bread, you will blossom, you'll avoid blood sugar and insulin spikes, your energy levels will even out, you'll prevent excessive fat storage, and your weight will drop.

Matthew Liebowitz, 14
High School Student

I think other teenagers could do it easily. There's always something to eat. If you like turkey sandwiches, you can eat hummus instead. If you like milk, you can have almond or rice milk. If you like sweets, you eat dark chocolate. If you like burgers, you get a meat substitute. If you like pizza, you get a cheeseless pizza with veggies.

There are a few things you have to be prepared for, like your friends will make fun of you. But I just make fun of them back. They say, "You can't eat like this every day, can you?" So I tell them, "Well, you can't eat meat every day, can you?" It's the same thing.

Week Two—Meat and Eggs

If it has a face or a mother, it has muscle, which always contains fat and cholesterol. Although red meat has more fat than chicken, most people don't know that they both contain about the same amount of cholesterol. Fish, meanwhile, which everyone is fond of for its healthy omega-3 fatty acids, can contain *more* cholesterol than either red meat or chicken. Steeped in saturated fat, cholesterol, and unhealthy animal protein, meat is left behind on the E2 Diet. Don't bother looking back.

Instead, explore the wonderful world of whole grains and legumes. Shop for rice, millet, oats, beans, barley, quinoa, wheat berries, whole wheat pasta, and whole wheat couscous.

Or try meat substitutes. Look into tofu (hard, medium, and soft), tempeh (a tasty fermented tofu), jackfruit (made from the world's largest treefruit, with the texture of pulled pork) wheat gluten (aka seitan), and some of the healthiest burgers and hot dogs made from plants. The E2 recipes (see Part III) will assist you in discovering and preparing new favorites.

TWO THINGS ARE WRONG with eggs: the yolk and the white. The yolk contains 212 milligrams of cholesterol and 5 grams of fat per egg. The white is almost pure animal protein, which is harsh on the kidneys and leaches calcium from your bones.

Be careful of using egg substitutes, too. Most of them contain egg white, or some other dairy product.

Week Three—Oil

Unlike most other plant-based diets, E2 asks you to do without added oils for the full four weeks—or at least a portion of them. When these weeks are over, you can reconsider oil, but I find that nearly everyone who goes oil-free likes it, and although they may add some oil back into their food, they discover that less is better.

Why is oil off-limits? Because the Engine 2 Diet is based on a whole food, nutrient-rich diet. Oil is certainly plant-based, whether it comes from olives, sunflowers, or corn, but it's not a whole food. The oil you buy in stores is extracted, meaning that the manufacturers take, say, a bunch of beautiful olives and, instead of leaving that oil in its wonderful natural package, squeeze out the good parts (healthy fiber, vitamins, and minerals). All that's left is the most refined and concentrated doses of calories on the planet—olive oil contains close to 4,100 calories per 16 ounces, or 120 calories per tablespoon! Oil's nutrient content is low, its saturated fat level is high, and all that fat goes straight to your waist and eventually clogs up your arteries.

Yes, olive oil is better than pure saturated fat because a large percentage of it is monounsaturated fat, which does seem to have health benefits. But 15 percent of olive oil is the saturated, artery-clogging kind. There are much better ways to get the healthier forms of fats than from refined and concentrated oils; instead, eat walnuts, ground flaxseed meal, soybeans, and green leafy vegetables.

WHY FOUR WEEKS?

Although the original Engine 2 Pilot Study lasted six weeks, I later discovered that its health benefits could often be achieved in as little as two.

The wonderful cholesterol results achieved by the participants at the three-week mark during the original Pilot Study inspired me to conduct a series of smaller studies, in which participants ate an all plant-based diet for only two weeks. These people achieved results comparable with those of the six-week study in every category except weight loss—naturally, the longer you are on this diet, the more weight you will lose.

Obviously, I am a big believer that the Engine 2 Diet is the best way to eat for life. However, my goal during the next four weeks is simply to let you experience how good it tastes to gain control of your palate, your weight, your lipids, and your health destiny. I know that you can accomplish all this in just four weeks while developing the skills, habits, and knowledge you'll need to increase your hunger to do even more.

And at the end of those four weeks, you'll find your body is a nutrient paradise. You will feel clean and light, energetic, and optimistic. And you will have accomplished this in less than a month!

Once those four weeks are over, you will face a big decision: Are you ready to commit to this lifestyle for additional weeks—or for the long term?

All the Engine 2 Pilot Study participants have decided to bring the Engine 2 Diet into their lives for good—but at different levels. Some are living it at 100 percent, some 95 percent, some 75 percent—and others are simply remembering to eat the healthy E2 way as often as possible.

What will you do? Will you be a 100 percenter? The more you continue living and eating this way, the easier it will get, making it difficult to return to your old dietary habits.

Or for lifestyle and personal reasons, maybe you will find it unrealistic to continue at the peak of the Engine 2 Diet, and will back off some of the time. Yet with even, say, a 75 percent commitment to the E2 Diet, you will still reap many of the benefits of living and eating this way.

BAD CHOICES/GOOD CHOICES

BAD	GOOD
Milk chocolate	70 percent cocoa dark chocolate (sparingly)
Chips and salsa	Toasted pita bread cut into pieces with salsa
Ice cream	Fruit sorbet
Mayonnaise	Homemade hummus spread or guacamole
Soda	Seltzer with a slice of fresh lemon or lime
Meat	Grilled marinated tofu, seitan, jackfruit, or tempeh
Hamburger/hot dog	Veggie burgers/hot dogs with all the trimmings
Cheese pizza	Nutritional yeast on whole grain pizza, ground-up nuts, sliced avocado—but go easy!
Cookies	Healthy fruit newtons, bananas rolled in finely chopped nuts

Or perhaps you will take a more flexitarian approach and simply make smart choices when pressed. Now that you know and understand the Engine 2 gold standard, you will bring a new awareness to your dietary choices: When you do eat meat or fish, you will choose wild salmon or skinless chicken breast; when you do eat dairy, you'll pick skim milk or nonfat yogurt/cheese. When you add oils, you'll go sparingly and avoid those high in saturated fats. And you'll eat primarily from the four healthy food groups: fruits, whole grains, vegetables, and legumes.

If at any point you feel as though your new eating habits and health are starting to slip away, find true north again. Repeat as much of the four-week diet as you can to recover your bearings. (The end-of-the-year holidays might be all it takes to throw you off-kilter. I know, I've been there.)

Marisa Pondo, 32
Child Caretaker

I used to buy nothing but meat and cheese. If I bought fruit, it was for margaritas. If I bought vegetables, it was for salsa. My idea of a good lunch was deep-frying a cheese sandwich. Then I decided to eat healthier, and to do that, I went E2. It changed my life. It's astonishing how much better I feel.

At first I was worried about money, but I've learned that I'm actually saving so much by doing this—$120 a month!

Experiment with what works best for you over the course of a year or two, and you'll be set for life.

E2 POP QUIZ

Q: If there are 4 grams of sugar in 1 teaspoon, and 39 grams of sugar in a 12-ounce can of Coca-Cola, how many teaspoons of sugar are in one can?

A: Each can of Coke contains 39 grams of sugar, or about 10 teaspoons full.

VICES AND VIRTUES

A good friend's father, a prominent neurosurgeon, always used to tell me, "If you have your health, you have everything." As a ten-year-old, I was clueless about that. It meant about as much as "the check is in the mail."

Now that I'm in my mid-fifties, his words make sense. Your health is one of your greatest assets. That is why, during your four weeks on the E2 Diet, I encourage you to go the extra mile and give up your unhealthy vices. It's worth it. Go whole hog. Jump in with both feet.

If you drink coffee, give it up, or switch to decaf. Same with tea. And if you don't give them up, remember not to add milk or cream. Instead, go for soy milk (look for the vitamin-fortified or the nonfat versions), or try various other nondairy substitutes, such as almond, oat, or rice milks.

You should restrict rich desserts, but you don't have to avoid sweets entirely. If you have a serious sweet tooth, try any of the Engine 2 dessert recipes or indulge in 70 percent or more dark chocolate. But avoid those egg- and cream-filled cakes!

I also encourage you to try giving up alcohol, at least for the full four weeks. Alcohol possesses no nutritional value, it inhibits your body's ability to burn fat by more than 30 percent, and it's loaded with empty calories. However, if you just can't go without, keep it down to one serving a day. Some recent evidence suggests that one glass of wine a day may even benefit your health—if you can limit it to one.

Remember, I am only talking about four weeks. The extent to which you stick with the program will determine your success at losing weight, lowering your cholesterol level, improving your gastrointestinal tract, and perfecting your overall health—as well as losing your cravings for the foods you thought you couldn't live without. At the end of the four-week period, you can return to your old habits if you wish. But my bet is the majority of you will continue down the pure path of healthy eating because you love the new-found you too much.

4

CRAZY MYTHS ABOUT FOOD

Jack LaLanne, the late vegetarian and fitness guru, recalled that when he started lifting weights in the 1930s, "The doctors were against me—they said that working out with weights would give people heart attacks and they would lose their sex drive."

Similarly, doctors didn't think smoking was bad for our health until the 1960s; in fact, they actually endorsed it until the 1950s. And there have been times when medical professionals thought cocaine was a legitimate medicine, when drilling a hole in the skull was considered a remedy for many diseases, and when a frontal lobotomy was thought to be sound therapy.

In many ways, things haven't changed. There's still a ton of misinformation out there, and much of it concerns plant-based eating. To make matters worse, doctors are seldom schooled in nutrition, and the ones who are tend to follow the antiquated food pyramid created by lobbyists and special-interest groups that are less interested in your health than in keeping their jobs and taking your money.

I can't believe all the incredible things I hear about diet and nutrition, spoken by people who don't have a clue but who talk as if they did. An all-protein diet is good for you! All carbs are terrible! God put animals on the planet for people to eat! Alcohol is a health tonic! Vegetarians are weak wusses who can't play sports!

So beware: Once you start eating the healthy, plant-based E2 way, people will begin to tell you all kinds of ridiculous "facts" about food. One course of action is to ignore them. But if you feel like getting into a debate, here's some information to help you shut 'em down.

Myth 1

You can't get enough protein eating a plant-based diet.

Reality: Not only will you get all the protein you need, for the first time in your life you won't suffer from an excess of it.

Ample amounts of protein are thriving in whole, natural plant-based foods. For example, spinach is 51 percent protein; mushrooms, 35 percent; beans, 26 percent; oatmeal, 16 percent; whole wheat pasta, 15 percent; corn, 12 percent; and potatoes, 11 percent.

What's more, our body needs less protein than you may think. According to the World Health Organization (WHO), the average 150-pound male requires only 50 grams of protein daily based on a 2,000 calorie a day diet, which means about 10 percent of calories should come from protein. Other nutritional organizations vary in their recommendations from as little as 2.5 percent of daily calories to 6 percent; most Americans, however, are taking in 20 percent or more.

Doctors from my father to Dean Ornish to Joel Fuhrman, author of the bestselling *Eat to Live: The Revolutionary Formula for Fast and Sustained Weight Loss* (Little, Brown), all suggest that getting an adequate amount of protein should be the least of your worries.

Look around you and tell me the last time you saw someone who was hospitalized for a protein deficiency. Or look around in nature, where you will notice that the largest and strongest animals, such as elephants, gorillas, hippos, and bison, are all plant eaters.

Also, the type of protein you consume is as important as the amount. If you are taking in most of your protein from animal-based foods, you're getting not only too much protein, but also an acid-producing form that wreaks havoc on your system.

Why is protein so potentially harmful? Because your body can store carbohydrates and fats, but not protein. So if the protein content of your diet exceeds the amount you need, not only will your liver and kidneys become overburdened, but you will start leaching calcium from your bones to neutralize the excess animal protein that becomes acidic in the human body.

That's why, in the case of protein, the adage "less is more" definitely applies. The average American consumes well over 100 grams daily—a dangerous amount. But if you eat a plant-strong diet, you'll be getting neither too much nor too little protein, but an amount that's just right.

Myth 2

Plant proteins aren't complete proteins.

Reality: Plant proteins are as complete as complete can be.

The myth that they're not, or are of a lesser quality than animal proteins, dates back to experiments performed on rats in the early 1900s. Forget the fact that rats aren't humans, have different nutritional requirements, and need more protein than humans to support their furry little bodies. The meat, dairy, and egg industries have marketed the hell out of this ancient research, and even in the year 2017 most every Dick, Tom, and Jane thinks the only way to get complete protein is through meat, eggs, or dairy.

In reality, proteins are composed of chains of roughly twenty different amino acids. Of those, eight are found outside our body and must be absorbed from our food. These eight are the "essential" amino acids. The remaining acids are "nonessential" because they can be synthesized by our bodies themselves.

Plants supply all the essential and nonessential amino acids. All of them. While some plants may be low in (not missing) one amino acid and other plants may be higher in another, your brilliant body sorts it all out and, at the end of the day, complements your amino-acid profile so it is perfectly balanced. In so doing, it creates a high-quality protein that is healthier, safer, and better than animal protein.

Thus, there is absolutely no need to combine certain plant proteins at each meal in an attempt to achieve an optimal amino acid balance.

Unfortunately, the protein-combination myth continues to be perpetuated by any number of respected organizations. But the Physicians Committee for Responsible Medicine gets it right. Its position statement reads: "A variety of grains, legumes, and vegetables can provide all of the essential amino acids our bodies require. It was once thought that various plant foods had to be eaten together to get their full protein value, otherwise known as protein combining or protein complementing. We now know that intentional combining is not necessary to obtain all of the essential amino acids. As long as the diet contains a variety of grains, legumes, and vegetables, protein needs are easily met."

Scream it from the mountaintops: Plant proteins are 100 percent complete!

Myth 3

Carbohydrates make us fat.

Reality: Some carbs do, but good carbs don't.

Most trendy diets claim that all carbohydrates are bad guys, yet of the three macronutrients that provide calories in our diet (carbs, protein, and fat), carbohydrates are the body's primary fuel source. They're responsible for managing your heart rate, digestion, breathing, exercising, walking, and thinking.

Roughly 70 percent of your daily calories should come from good (complex) carbohydrates. The ones to avoid are called simple carbs.

Both types of carbs are sugars. Both are digested and converted into glucose, which is used by the body for energy: in the blood as glucose, or stored in either the muscles or the liver as glycogen. When consumed in excess, carbohydrates can be converted to fat.

Simple carbohydrates include table sugar, molasses, honey, alcohol, white bread, white pasta, white rice, fried chips, sugary cereals, fruit juices, candy, and milk. Most simple carbs are nutritionally empty because they have been tinkered with by humans, stripped of their fiber, minerals, and vitamins. They are digested quickly by the body and cause a sharp spike in your blood sugar levels.

In response to this spike, your pancreas pumps out insulin to transport and deliver the energy-bearing glucose to cells throughout your body. This process causes your blood sugar and insulin levels to swing like a pendulum, leaving you feeling fatigued, hungry, and craving still more simple carbohydrates.

And because simple carbohydrates are digested so quickly, any excess sugar is converted to fat. For these reasons, most simple carbohydrates are a poor food choice.

In contrast, complex carbohydrates are nutritious, and include vegetables, whole grain breads and pastas, beans, peas, brown rice, sweet potatoes, oats, fruits, and whole grain cereals. They are loaded with fiber, vitamins, minerals, and micronutrients. Unlike simple carbohydrates, complex carbohydrates cause a balanced and controlled release of sugar into your system. This slow release gives the body more time to use the carbohydrates as fuel; as a result, fewer turn to fat and insulin remains stable.

So if you consume whole, good, natural carbs, you will enjoy more consistent energy throughout the day without gaining extra pounds.

As you can see, the two types of carbs differ immensely from a nutritional standpoint. Simple carbohydrates are calorie laden, providing little nutrition and causing weight gain. Complex carbohydrates are lower in calories and, because they are loaded with fiber, provide bulk that fills you up sooner, alleviates hunger pangs, and keeps you feeling satisfied longer.

So go eat your carbs—as long as they're complex.

Myth 4

You can't get enough calcium eating a plant-based diet.

Reality: A diverse, plant-based diet is one of the best available sources of calcium—and lets you avoid the deleterious effects associated with dairy products.

Great sources of calcium include green leafy vegetables, nuts, oranges, kidney beans, lima beans, whole grains, Swiss chard, lentils, raisins, broccoli, kale, celery, tofu, and romaine lettuce.

One reason why Americans have such a high incidence of osteoporosis (or weakening of the bones) isn't a lack of dietary calcium but an excess of animal protein, which leaches calcium from the bones.

In fact, did you know that the countries with the highest rate of dairy consumption, including the United States, New Zealand, Britain, and Sweden, also have the highest rates of osteoporosis? Although their citizens consume massive amounts of dietary calcium, the excessive protein in that milk, cheese, steak, fish, and eggs always trumps this important mineral, leaving them with a net deficit.

Meanwhile, people in rural China, who consume one-third the amount of dairy we do, have almost zero cases of osteoporosis. Dr. John McDougall, author of *The McDougall Program for a Healthy Heart,* has scoured the medical literature on the topic and has yet to find one case of dietary calcium deficiency in humans—so long as they consumed an adequate number of calories. So no milk mustache for you!

Myth 5

You can't get enough fat eating a plant-based diet.

Reality: Trace amounts of fat are present in all fruits, vegetables, and other plant foods.

Strawberries are 5 percent fat; bell peppers, 6 percent; broccoli, 8 percent; spinach, 11 percent; and soybeans, 41 percent. Several high-fat plant foods contain in excess of 80 percent fat, including certain nuts and seeds, as well as avocados, olives, and coconuts.

By eating a delicious, plant-happy diet, you will consume roughly 9 to 15 percent of your total calories from fat, which is ideal.

Getting your fat from plant-based foods means you will be consuming healthy monounsaturated and polyunsaturated fats as opposed to dangerous saturated fats. You will be able to eat more food than you ever dreamed of without gaining weight, and feel wonderful.

Myth 6

You can't be a competitive athlete and eat plants.

Reality: Tell that to Tony Gonzalez, the 247-pound former tight end for the Kansas City Chiefs and the Atlanta Falcons. For health reasons, Tony changed his diet after signing a five-year contract extension, making him the NFL's highest-paid tight end, and went on to break the league record for receptions by a tight end in 2008. His teammates have nicknamed him *China*

James Garee, 25
Firefighter

Before becoming a firefighter, I was co-captain of the University of Colorado football team, where I weighed three hundred pounds. To keep up my weight, I used to eat 8,000 calories a day—I'd go to Arby's and ask for five Arby meals, an order of curly fries, and a large Coke. But ever since Rip flipped me, I've lost over sixty pounds. But it can be difficult. Food is personal. If you don't understand what someone is eating, you go into a kind of defense meltdown. For example, if you tell people that the way they eat at home isn't good for them, they'll say, "Are you telling me that my granny's trying to poison me?"

Study after T. Colin Campbell's book of the same name, which Gonzalez studied before changing his diet—and which you will soon be reading about.

Or tell that to Ruth Heidrich, who in 1982 was diagnosed with metastatic breast cancer and cured herself by eating a low-fat, plant-strong diet. She has since won more than one thousand triathlons. Or tell Salim Stoudamire, the plant-eating former point guard for the NBA Atlanta Hawks, who says that by the fourth quarter, when most players are starting to fade, he was picking it up a notch. Or tell Martina Navratilova, the world's winningest tennis player, who served up plant-based foods during the height of her career. Or tell Dave Scott, one of my heroes and six-time winner of the famed Hawaii Ironman triathlon, who was a known plant-devourer at his peak.

Or better yet, try going plant-based yourself and see how much your own athletic performance improves.

Myth 7

By eating only plant-based foods, you'll miss key nutrients.

Reality: You'll be stockpiling away the nutrients like never before, improving your health, and reversing disease. If you were to hold a triathlon based on the quantity of nutrients in each food, plants would cross the finish line and get a massage before meat, dairy, and eggs even had a chance to get off the bicycle.

Calorie for calorie, the most nutrient-dense foods are plants, not animals. After all, plants are the mother source of all calories and all nutrients for all creatures, whereas animal-based foods are essentially plant foods recycled into an unhealthy package.

The only nutrient that plant-based foods lack is vitamin B12. But you can get a daily supply of B12 by downing two tablespoons of nutritional yeast, a glass of fortified soy milk, a bowl of fortified cereal, or, if you wish, a daily 500-microgram pill that should be chewed or dissolved in the mouth to increase absorption.

Myth 8

If you eat only plant-based food, your energy will be low.

Reality: Your energy levels will be more constant and consistent than at any other point in your life.

Think of high-fiber and nutrient-heavy plant foods as the big logs in the fireplace that burn for hours. Think of low-fiber and nutrient-light foods such as simple carbohydrates as wads of newspaper that go up in a flash. When you're eating plant-strong, you won't have the energy peaks and valleys of the past, and if you so choose, you won't even need coffee to get your butt and mind in gear in the mornings. You'll awake feeling refreshed, even-keeled, and excited about charging forward into your day.

Myth 9

A plant-based diet is bad for children and pregnant mothers.

Reality: By the age of two (once off mother's milk), every child is ready for a plant-strong diet. Even renowned expert Dr. Benjamin Spock recommended the practice in the seventh edition of his classic bestselling book, *Baby and Child Care*, the last edition published before his death at ninety-four. If you start them young, your kids will develop a palate that appreciates the subtleties of plant foods and will gain the healthy rewards that accompany this diet as they grow.

Pregnant women, meanwhile, can get all the vitamins, nutrients, and minerals that both they and their babies need to be healthy and well. My wife, Jill, ate an all-plant-based diet throughout her three pregnancies with no morning sickness and no complications.

Myth 10

Everyone needs to take fish oil supplements to ensure they're getting essential omega-3 fatty acids.

Reality: There are numerous ways to get essential omega-3 fatty acids without subjecting yourself to the potential risks of fish oils—which, according to the Physicians Committee for Responsible Medicine, are highly unstable molecules that can break down and release dangerous, disease-causing free radicals.

People are under the false assumption that taking a fish oil supplement will negate the effects of all the cheese, meat, and processed foods they throw down their throats. But fish oil is no panacea. It can actually raise total and LDL cholesterol levels, increases your chance of a hemorrhagic stroke, and suppresses the immune system.

Instead of taking fish oil, rely on ground flaxseed meal, walnuts, soybeans, and green leafy vegetables, all of which contain plenty of essential omega-3 fatty acids.

If you are unwilling to transition to a totally plant-strong diet, then go to a health food store and buy some plant-based omega-3 supplements that come straight from the mother source: plankton from the oceans, seas, and lakes—which, by the way, is where fish get their omega-3s.

Myth 11

Real men don't eat plants.

Reality: The fat and cholesterol in animal products clogs up the arteries traveling not only to the heart and head but also to the extremities, including the penis, where they can cause PAD (peripheral arterial disease) and impotence, which research shows may be an early sign of heart disease.

So, men: There is a better way, and it doesn't involve taking Viagra, Cialis, or Levitra. It involves eating fruits, vegetables, whole grains, and beans.

In my father's research study, several of the men who had been impotent for years regained their performance after changing to a plant-based diet, making their wives quite happy. Many of the Engine 2 Pilot Study participants also reported improved potency, including one who said that his erections "are now like blue steel."

Myth 12

Eating plant-based foods is joyless.

Reality: Plant-based foods are delicious and satisfying.

The longer you're on the E2 Diet, the more your palate will change. Think about milk, for instance. Since it's well known that whole milk is not good for you, you've probably cut back to 2 percent or skim. At first, I bet that skim milk tasted like water. Then you became accustomed to it so when you tried whole milk again, it tasted like liquid paint. Your palate had changed.

It's the same with adding oil to your foods. Anthony Salerno, one of the E2 Pilot Study participants, is a fourth-generation Italian-American who thought he couldn't live without his olive oil. But after six weeks on the E2 Diet, he found he enjoyed meals more without it—the oil, he realized, disguised their true flavors. When he returned to using olive oil, he found it tasted as though he'd poured synthetic goo on his food.

Brandon and Amy Marsh, 32, 29
Triathletes

Even though we're triathletes, we never paid much attention to our diets. But when Rip was looking for volunteers for the Engine 2 Pilot Study, we signed up—and it worked. After all, we pay attention to everything else we do for our bodies, why shouldn't we also be paying attention to everything we eat? The fact is, sometimes your performance can start with your fork. Diet counts as much as training.

Foods taste better without being dunked in butter, drenched in margarine, or saturated with sour cream. Plant-based foods are absolutely glorious in their sublimeness. Without all the extra fat and processed flavors drowning them out, you'll finally get to taste nuances you might never have noticed: the tang of a ripe red bell pepper, the zest of a cara cara orange, or the zing of a plate of lacinato kale with roasted garlic—foods bursting with flavors all their own.

5

THE MEDICAL PROOF BEHIND THE ENGINE 2 DIET

As a firefighter, I saw the adverse effects of poor diet every day on the job—because all firefighters in Austin are also EMTs (emergency medical technicians).

Firefighters are EMTs because more than 70 percent of our calls aren't fires but medical emergencies. Approximately another 15 to 20 percent are car accidents, spills, and alarm activations. These statistics mean that if the city of Austin has 100,000 calls a year, around 70,000 of them are medical related.

To become an EMT, we have to attend a two-month mini–medical school during our fire academy training. We learn how to handle myriad accidents as well as to treat various acute illnesses such as cardiac and respiratory arrest, heart attacks, strokes, seizures, diabetic emergencies, respiratory problems, and traumatic injuries including falls, fractures, lacerations, stabbings, burns, and sprains. We're also taught how to perform a complete patient assessment and to obtain a medical history.

On a regular basis we conduct procedures such as cardiopulmonary resuscitation (CPR) and artificial ventilation; administering oxygen and performing basic airway management (to make sure victims are breathing properly); bandaging and splinting; and dispensing medicines, such as aspirin and nitroglycerin (in two forms, one as a pill placed under the tongue, the other as a chest paste). We administer glucose for diabetic emergencies, epinephrine for allergic reactions, and albuterol in case of a severe asthma attack.

The reason we go on so many medical calls is that, nine times out of ten, we can arrive on the scene several minutes before Emergency Medical Services (EMS) shows up: Austin has forty-four fire stations compared with twenty-eight EMS stations, and sometimes the difference between saving and losing a life can be a matter of mere seconds.

Of course, when I first joined the department, I imagined we'd go racing out to a big fire at least once a shift. I saw myself as a character in the movie *The Towering Inferno*—climbing up fifty flights of stairs and then coming down carrying little old ladies on my back, or scurrying commando-style on my hands and knees under the smoke, finding a child under a bed, handing him out the window to my partner at the top of a twenty-four-foot extension ladder, then flying out a window onto a trampoline.

The reality is that we can go a month without seeing a single fire, then see two fires in one shift. They cycle in and out with no rhyme or reason. Yet while fighting fires is a very inconsistent part of our job, making medical calls has become very predictable.

Why? Because Americans are in dire need of emergency medical assistance. So instead of fighting fires, we fight the battle for America's health. And there appears to be no end in sight to this battle.

Take a long hard look around you. Do you see what I see? Americans are downing empty calories with reckless abandon, gorging on vats of animal-based products teeming with unhealthy fat, cholesterol, and acid-producing protein; gobbling up refined and processed foods; drizzling, swathing, and dumping concentrated vegetable oils into, over, and through everything and anything without thinking twice.

We've become addicted to the taste, texture, and comfort these foods give us. But unfortunately, what they also give us is a breeding ground for the ailments and diseases that are tearing at the seams of our nation's health. High blood pressure is the norm. Constipation and irritable bowel syndrome are commonplace. Migraine headaches—and headaches in general—bring tears to our eyes. Osteoporosis is breaking us down. PMS, allergies, infections, and eczema have increased in frequency and intensity. Kidney stones and gallstones are more than a pain in the side.

All these conditions are influenced by a poor diet, and they add up to a big mess. However, the crowning blow to American health is the lineup of killer diseases taking us down like rows of dominoes: heart disease, cancer, stroke, diabetes, obesity, and Alzheimer's disease.

Yet there is hope—in the form of a great deal of scientific evidence showing that a plant-healthy diet can prevent, and even reverse, most of these diseases.

You now know how to respond to those who can't tell a myth from reality. Read on if you really want to show people that you know the hard science behind why you're eating so healthily and happily.

HEART DISEASE

Twelve years ago, at 10:06 p.m., a call came in from the White Swan Lounge and Bar on Austin's east side. LD Davis, the owner and proprietor, had suffered a heart attack.

When we arrived, LD wasn't breathing and had no pulse. One of the patrons had already started doing chest compressions; we thanked her, dived in, and started doing them ourselves.

Next, we took out a BVM (or bag valve mask, which allows firefighters to breathe for patients without putting our mouths over theirs), and placed it over LD's mouth and nose. The task can be tricky, because the patient's tongue frequently falls back into his or her throat, blocking the airway. To prevent that, we often have to use an oropharyngeal airway, a curved, straw-like device that keeps the tongue in place.

We worked on LD as a team. One of us performed chest compressions and another held down the mouthpiece to ensure that no air could escape, and I squeezed the bag part of the BVM with both hands at a slow and steady rate of roughly ten squeezes per minute. A fourth firefighter made sure oxygen was hooked up to the BVM, took out the AED (a machine called an automated external defibrillator), checked for vital signs (heart rate and breathing), and alternated doing chest compressions with us.

While all this was going on, the bar's patrons formed a semicircle around us, chanting, "Come on, LD, you can make it!" I got goose bumps all over my body, and was chanting as well: "Come on, LD!"

We placed the pads from the AED on LD's chest, powered it up, and waited a few seconds while it analyzed his heart, looking for a shockable rhythm. The machine works when the heart is in a state of what's called ventricular fibrillation. At that point, we can shock the patient in the hope of rebooting the heart's proper rhythm.

We did find a shockable rhythm, so we shocked LD—with no results. So we continued CPR.

By this time, EMS had arrived and set up an IV (intravenous line). They also gave LD some drugs to assist in restarting his heart. Again we tried shocking him, again with no luck. However, on the third attempt we were successful. The crowd cheered and celebrated. Two of us then rode in the back of the ambulance and continued breathing for LD until we arrived at the hospital and handed him off to the emergency room doctors.

I later heard from the EMS crew that LD was up and about again; he managed to live for another year and a half before dying—from another heart attack.

Whenever we firefighters are able to bring people back to life from what looks like certain death, the department presents us with a Phoenix Award, named for the mythological bird that rose from the ashes after dying in flames. Over the course of my career I've received three Phoenixes, all for helping patients who had suffered heart attacks. I'm proud of them, but wish my skills hadn't been needed.

LD's STORY IS FAR FROM UNIQUE. Heart disease kills more Americans than the next four fatal diseases combined. Close to one million of us die of cardiac complications annually, and one in every two Americans will die from heart disease or stroke.

This illness has gained traction over the last century—in 1900, cardiovascular disease wasn't even in the top ten causes of death. By 2014, though, one person every 53 second was dying from heart disease each and every day.

Dr. Lewis Kuller of the University of Pittsburgh reported the ten-year findings of the Cardiovascular Health Study, a project of the National Heart, Lung, and Blood Institute. Its conclusion: All males older than sixty-five and females older than seventy who have been exposed to the traditional Western diet are already suffering from cardiovascular disease and should be treated as such.

Even more frightening: In more than half of all heart disease cases, the first symptom is instant death.

What is at the core of this terrible disease? Plaque. Plaque is a waxy, fatty deposit that can build up in various places in the body, including the inside of the arteries.

There are two types of plaque formations: large, hardened, stable ones; and small, soft, unstable ones.

Extensive buildup of the larger plaques within the arteries limits the amount of oxygen-rich blood the heart receives. This process can cause angina, or severe discomfort and pain in the chest region. Patients with angina are often prescribed nitroglycerin pills, which dilate (open up and relax) the arteries, allowing the heart to receive more blood. At other times the narrowing of the arteries due to plaque can completely shut off the blood supply and cause a heart attack.

Most people believe that the larger blockages are the primary cause of heart attacks; actually, they represent only 10 percent of all cases. Why? Because over the course of many years, the miraculous human body compensates for plaque blockages by creating new channels that reroute blood around them, similar to the way a river might redirect itself around a large boulder. Eventually, the plaques form scar tissue and calcify, making them stable. The other 90 percent of heart attacks are caused by the small, soft plaques, which are less than 50 percent of the width of the artery. These obnoxious rascals appear when your blood and the endothelium, or the silky smooth lining of your arteries, become sticky. This tackiness permits lethal LDL cholesterol to attach and burrow into the artery wall.

To heal this injury, the body forms the equivalent of a pimple, inside of which certain enzymes act to weaken its cover, making it delicate as a cobweb. The blood flowing past eventually causes the pimple to burst.

Next, the natural blood-clotting platelets in your blood rush to heal the injury, a clot rapidly develops and enlarges, preventing any blood from flowing downstream to the heart. Bam! You have a heart attack.

So how do you prevent the formation of these terrible plaques? Stop eating animal-based products!

Animal-based products contain all the building blocks for heart disease: artery-clogging saturated fat, plaque-promoting dietary cholesterol, cholesterol-raising and inflammation-causing animal protein, and free-radical-promoting oxidants. All these components encourage the buildup of plaque and damage the silky lining of the sixty-thousand-plus miles of arteries, veins, and capillaries through which your blood flows.

Plant-based products discourage plaque buildup and promote the health of your artery lining because they contain healthy unsaturated fats, zero cholesterol, friendly protein, and free-radical-zapping antioxidants. And unlike animal-based products, plants are nutritional powerhouses, with the ability to prevent and even reverse existing heart disease. Plants are loaded with vitamins, minerals, phytochemicals, and bioflavonoids.

Why am I so confident of the connection between diet and heart disease? Because so many studies have proven that heart disease need never exist, and that existing heart disease can be halted in its tracks, or even reversed.

As mentioned, my father, Dr. Caldwell B. Esselstyn, Jr., conducted the most profound evidence-based research on the arrest and reversal of heart disease on the planet; his patients demonstrated striking reversal of the plaque in their diseased arteries.

Remember his prescription? Eat a completely low-fat, plant-based diet.

My father was not the only person to show a reversal of heart disease. For example, just as my father was embarking on his arrest and reversal study, Dr. Dean Ornish was also conducting his second Lifestyle Heart Trial study at the University of California at San Francisco, whose results were published in the medical journal *The Lancet.*

Ornish worked with two groups of patients stricken with heart disease. For one year, a group of twenty-eight individuals ate a pure plant-based diet supplemented with moderate exercise and a stress-management program. At the same time, a control group of twenty patients consumed the typical American diet.

The outcome: The patients on the low-fat, plant-based diet saw a reversal in, or an end to, their preexisting coronary blockages, as well as a reduction in or elimination of their angina. However, the members of the standard American diet control group saw an increase in their coronary blockages, as well as in the frequency and intensity of their angina.

What caused these results? First, by avoiding all animal-based products, the plant-eating patients eliminated all the major building blocks that contribute to plaque formation: fat, cholesterol, and animal protein. They were able to lower their total cholesterol to a level that helped their body metabolize away the plaque buildup in their arteries.

Second, by consuming only fresh fruits, vegetables, whole grains, and legumes, the patients allowed the arteries themselves to heal at a cellular and metabolic level. A plant-based diet permits the silky lining of the arteries to produce nitric oxide, an element crucial to their health that cleans the blood, heals the endothelium (making it slippery instead of sticky), and allows the capillaries, arteries, and veins to relax, letting more blood flow to the heart.

Corroborating this research, in 2004 Cornell professor Dr. T. Colin Campbell, the project director of the China-Oxford-Cornell Diet and Health Project, published *The China Study*, a book chronicling the results of a thirty-year investigation of nutrition and health that examined more than 6,500 people in sixty-five different Chinese villages. *The New York Times* referred to this study as the "Grand Prix" of all epidemiological research.

Among the study's findings: American men are seventeen times more likely to die from heart disease than rural Chinese men. During one three-year period in the study, Campbell even found certain areas in China with populations over 100,000 where not a single person under the age of sixty-five had died from heart disease.

All of the Chinese subjects ate a predominantly whole food, plant-based diet, containing few to no packaged products (or meals at restaurants). As a result, their average total cholesterol ranged between 81 and 135.

Conversely, the typical American eats an animal-based diet with close to 40 percent of his or her calories coming from animal products, 50 percent from refined and processed sources, and only 10 percent from plant foods. Not surprisingly, Americans, who also rely heavily on packaged food products, have an average total cholesterol of 215.

The Framingham Heart Study, the largest equivalent review of diet and heart disease among Americans, had results similar to those of *The China Study*.

The Framingham study was initiated because heart disease had become so prevalent in this country during the last century that, in 1948, researchers from the National Institutes of Health (NIH) began what has become the longest ongoing investigation into the causes of heart disease ever conducted.

After compiling data on almost everyone in the entire town of Framingham, Massachusetts, the NIH researchers were able to determine that the leading risk factors for heart disease were (1) high cholesterol levels, (2) high blood pressure, and (3) cigarette smoking.

Further research over the last half century has confirmed these findings. Today, a high cholesterol level is still the number one risk factor for heart disease, greater than smoking, high blood pressure, family history, stress, or obesity.

Interestingly, nobody in the Framingham Study whose total cholesterol level was under 150 without using cholesterol-lowering drugs ever had a heart attack. Once again, as Dr. William Castelli, the former director of the Framingham Study, puts it: Keep your total cholesterol under 150 and you protect yourself from ever having a heart attack.

And get this! Some 35 percent of all heart attacks documented in the Framingham Study occurred in people whose total cholesterol level was between 151 and 200, numbers the American Heart Association and most physicians will tell you are rock solid.

This research indicates that the only way to become truly rock solid is to get your total cholesterol below 150 and your LDL cholesterol below 80. You can best do this by eating a delicious plant-based diet.

The sooner you can start, the better off you'll be. For example, autopsies of young American soldiers from the Korean and Vietnam Wars confirmed that 80 percent already had plaque deposits greater than 50 percent of the width of their coronary arteries, while the Korean and Vietnamese soldiers examined, who had eaten a plant-based diet, had little to no plaque.

We also know from the landmark PDAY (Pathobiological Determinants of Atherosclerosis in Youth) Study, begun in 1985 and supported by the NIH's National Heart, Lung, and Blood Institute, that adolescents who died from accidents, homicides, and suicides already had the makings of fatty plaque lesions in their coronary arteries. In other words, dangerous levels can build up long before you hit the age most people associate with heart attacks.

STROKE

Stroke is a silent killer that hits like a well-camouflaged assassin perched in a tree. Stroke attacks with no warning signs, and results in death 25 percent of the time. Of every five people who die of stroke, three are women and two are men. Nearly 800,000 Americans suffer strokes annually, and 130,000 of these victims die.

A stroke is similar to a heart attack, but affects the brain. It can occur in one of two ways. The first type, called ischemic stroke, is the result of a blood clot, or a narrowing of the arteries to the brain.

The second type, hemorrhagic stroke, occurs when one of the arteries leading to the brain ruptures. In both cases, there isn't enough oxygen-rich blood feeding and nourishing the brain. Nerve cells in the brain then die, affecting the part of the body those cells controlled.

Strokes range from ministrokes called TIAs (transient ischemic attacks) lasting from one to twenty-four hours, to full-blown strokes causing complete paralysis or death.

Stroke and heart disease are both diseases of the cardiovascular system. As with heart disease, in a stroke your vessels (another term for capillaries, arteries, and veins) can't keep pace with the massive quantities of fat, grease, and cholesterol you consistently ask them to process. Plaque deposits start to accumulate until you develop either large, stable plaques, which cause narrowing of the arteries, or the small, delicate ones that rupture and cause a clot.

Keeping your blood pressure in check can minimize stroke risk—but eating meat, dairy, eggs, and added oils raises blood pressure in several ways. First, narrowed and clogged vessels require an increase in pressure to circulate blood throughout the body. Second, the saturated fat in meat and dairy makes the blood thicker, which again requires an increase in pressure to move it through the body. Third, animal products are notoriously high in sodium, causing the body and blood to retain fluid, which again causes an increase in blood pressure.

Americans consume far too much sodium, not only from animal-based products but also from canned and packaged goods and restaurant meals. Instead, we should be increasing our intake of potassium, a mineral that removes sodium from the blood and, in turn, reduces blood pressure. This is why stroke expert Dr. Mitchell Elkind of Columbia University's Department of Neurology suggests that to reduce stroke, people should "eat a diet rich in fruits and vegetables high in potassium, along with a low-fat, low-sodium diet."

According to the Framingham Study, for every three additional servings of fruits and vegetables you eat a day, the risk of stroke is reduced by 22 percent. And according to a ten-year study presented at the 1993 meeting of the American Heart Association, female survivors of strokes or heart attacks could cut their future stroke risk by eating spinach, carrots, and other fruits and vegetables containing vitamins C, E, and B2 and beta-carotene.

(Vitamin C is present in many foods, including citrus fruits, bell peppers, and kale. Vitamin B2, or riboflavin, and vitamin E can be found in green leafy vegetables and nuts, as well as in many other plant-based foods. Beta-carotene is a form of vitamin A present in fruits and vegetables.)

So be proactive. Eat a whole food, nutrient-rich, plant-based diet. Never allow the building blocks of stroke and heart disease—artery-clogging saturated fat, dietary cholesterol, and acidic animal protein—into your body.

Stroke can hit anyone at any time. For example, I can remember when my grandfather, the great doctor Barney Crile, suffered a stroke in his late seventies. He was standing in his kitchen when he suddenly fell over backward and landed on one of his two cats, Sunday Morning in the Twilight Gleaming (a crazy-pills long name for a cat the size of a dog). The cat came out of it fine, but Barney wasn't as lucky. He had partial paralysis to the left side of his body and his quick wit and brilliant mind were dulled.

I am confident Barney could have avoided his stroke if he hadn't been such a lover of dining on all things animal. He was a madman when it came to eating anything and everything. He would jump out of the car when he saw fresh road kill, scoop it up, take it home, skin it, and incorporate it into the family dinner. A menu of ten different meals that hung on the kitchen wall epitomized the Crile eating style. First on the list: bear balls roasted in bacon fat.

Don't eat bear balls. Eat healthy, delectable, plant-based foods so that you will never fall over on your cat.

CANCER

Cancer. The C word. It fans fear in the hearts of Americans. And rightfully so. Cancer is the second-leading cause of death each year and, according to the American Hospital Association, will surpass the number one cause, heart disease, within five years. One in every three people will contract cancer in their lifetime, and one in four will die from it.

Cancer can be ruthless and take you down in a matter of months. Cancer can be relentless and drag on for decades. Cancer often requires surgery, which can be disfiguring and painful. Cancer causes depression, with its energy-zapping chemotherapy and radiation treatments. Cancer is horrific.

Cancer is everywhere. Take a look around you and you will see how it has blemished almost every family in America—including the families of our firefighters at the station: Steve Martinez's father died at fifty-two of colorectal cancer, James Garee's father died at fifty-seven of lung cancer, and Scottie Walters' seventy-one-year-old father endured chemotherapy for throat cancer.

How does this menace start? At the cellular level. Each of us has billions of cells in our body. For the most part, these cells are programmed to grow, divide, and then die.

Cancer begins when normal cells mutate and become abnormal due to various environmental, nutritional, or chemical stresses. They then start to grow and divide wildly, refusing to die, doubling every one hundred days—and yet it can take ten to fifteen years before such cancers reach the size of a match tip.

Eventually these renegade cells clump together to form a tumor, killing off healthy tissue as it competes for space and blood vessels to acquire nutrients. Parts of the tumor can even break away, spread throughout the body, and start other tumors. This process, called metastasis, is usually a death sentence.

But you can lower your cancer risk. Like heart disease, cancer loses its power if you don't feed it the things it craves to flourish—dairy, meat, eggs, oils, processed sugar, tobacco, and alcohol.

Even if you already have cancer, you can reduce its growth by lessening your reliance on animal foods and reaching for plant foods.

Let's explore why, starting with dairy products. Multiple studies show that dairy products contain cancer-promoting saturated fat; animal protein; and insulin-like growth factor-1 (IGF-1), a powerful growth-promoting hormone and known cancer culprit.

Saturated fat suppresses the immune system and contains excessive calories, which spur growth of all cells—even cancer cells. According to *The China Study*'s T. Colin Campbell, the animal protein in dairy foods (even fat-free products) contributes to an acidic environment in which cancer cells and tumors thrive.

As for IGF-1, this substance actually changes our hormonal balance, according to Dr. John McDougall. In women, IGF-1 can increase estrogen levels, known to promote breast and ovarian cancer, and in men, it can increase testosterone levels, known to promote testicular and prostate cancers.

In fact, a June 1999 article in the journal *Alternative Medicine Reviews* reported that prostate cancer was more strongly correlated with the consumption of nonfat dairy products than with any other food product.

Let's remember where all dairy comes from—the cow. Cow's milk is 20 percent protein if it's whole (40 percent if it's skim), most of which comes from casein—a dairy protein shown to be a tumor promoter. Furthermore, the amount of fat in milk averages around 50 percent, a large percentage of which is saturated. The remaining 35 percent of milk's calories come from the carbohydrate milk lactose, to which 70 percent of the world is intolerant.

Cow's milk is fine for a calf who wants to gain one thousand pounds in less than a year. Whenever possible, humans should stick to breast milk until the age of two, and then make the switch to a milk substitute.

Meat is another problem. Meat protein creates an acidic environment that is also a breeding ground for cancer cells and growth hormones. And meat fat is a magnet for chemical carcinogens that are stored in fat tissue—fiends such as mercury, dioxin, PCBs (polychlorinated biphenyls), and DDT.

Meat is also high in oxidants, such as iron, which not only oxidize cholesterol—a process that makes it more easily deposited in your arteries—but also promotes free radicals that mutate your cells' DNA and turn them into renegade cancer cells.

To top it all off, meat, with its lack of fiber, stalls fecal matter in the colon for extended periods of time, which in turn can contribute to colon cancer.

An eight-year study conducted in conjunction with the American Association of Retired Persons that followed more than 500,000 people between the ages of fifty and seventy-one showed that people who frequently eat meat have a higher risk of several types of cancer—including lung, colorectal, esophageal, liver, and pancreatic—than people who don't.

As for eggs, these devils are not as incredible and edible as the egg industry wants you to believe. As mentioned, the yolk contains more than 200 milligrams of cholesterol, while the white is one of the most concentrated sources of animal protein around. And you now know the dangers of animal protein.

A twenty-year study of diet and ovarian cancer published in *The Journal of the American Medical Association* showed that women who ate eggs three or more days each week "had a three times greater risk of fatal ovarian cancer than did women who ate eggs less than one day per week."

Oils, even so-called heart-healthy olive oil, are another debacle. Oil is fat. As noted earlier, all vegetable oils are 100 percent fat and are the most concentrated source of calories on the planet: 120 per tablespoon. Fat, whatever its form—monounsaturated, polyunsaturated, or saturated—is loaded with almost 10 calories per gram. Study after study has shown that when the percentage of fat calories in the diet exceeds 15 percent of caloric intake, cancer starts to rear its ugly head.

Sugar is yet another mess. Cancer cells swarm to sugar like bees to honey, because it is an important source of food for them. So the farther you stay away from packaged candies, sugary cereals, sodas, juice drinks, refined grains, and alcohol, the better. Instead, swarm to the good sugars found in fruits, vegetables, beans, and whole grains.

Kin Gill, 41
Lawyer

On Rip's diet, I've lost about eleven pounds, my cholesterol dropped 30 points, and my body fat fell 10 percent. One of the other great things about the diet is that it's a socially responsible way to eat. You're being more sensitive to animals, to the environment. You're not putting a lot of methane out to keep the feedlots going, you can focus on locally grown produce.

Enough about cancer promotion. Now let's look at cancer prevention.

More than thirty years ago, Dr. John McDougall published the first study showing that women can treat breast cancer successfully without surgery, chemotherapy, or drugs by making the switch from an animal-based diet to a nutrient-dense, plant-based diet.

Along the same lines, Dr. Dean Ornish completed a study in 1994 showing that nutritional intervention could halt, and even reverse, the progress of early-stage prostate cancer.

Ornish's study involved ninety-three men with prostate cancer; for one year, he put half of them on a low-fat, plant-based diet, and half on the standard American diet. He also took blood tests to measure before and after levels of their PSA. PSA, or prostate-specific antigen, is a protein produced by the cells of the prostate gland; levels can be used to detect tumors. Anything over 4.0 ng/ml (nanograms of PSA per milliliter) is considered elevated.

At the start of the study, all of the men had PSA levels between 4.0 and 10.0 ng/ml. The men eating the low-fat, plant-based diet saw a 4 percent decrease in their PSA, while those in the control group (eating the American diet) had a 6 percent increase. Powerful results!

In another study involving men with prostate cancer (this one from 2008), Dr. Ornish was able to show how disease-promoting genes can be turned off and disease-preventing ones turned on. After following a plant-healthy diet for just three months, the study participants were able to change the activity in close to 500 genes—with more than 453 turned off and 48 turned on. The takeaway message: It's not all in the genes, it's in the food!

T. Colin Campbell has also shown that while cancers and tumors in laboratory mice thrive on animal protein, plant protein almost repels cancer. Why? As discussed, animal proteins are acidic, creating an ideal environment in which cancer cells can thrive; plant proteins are alkaline, making it almost impossible for cancer cells to take root and prosper.

Campbell's recommendation: "The more you substitute plant foods for animal foods the healthier you are likely to be. I now consider an all plant-based diet the ideal diet for optimal health and to reduce disease risk."

DESPITE ALL THE EVIDENCE—and what I've described is just the proverbial tip of the iceberg—America has yet to hear and fully digest the plant-based message. As a result, the overall incidence of cancer has increased dramatically.

In fact, a plant-based diet possesses an arsenal of ingredients that help the body ward off cancer at a cellular and biochemical level: namely fiber, phytochemicals, and antioxidants. A plant-based diet contains many different types of fiber that drag toxins and carcinogens through the intestines and out of the body while keeping your bowel movements regular. A plant-based diet contains more than 12,000 phytochemicals, which ward off disease, increase the body's immune defenses, and slow down the aging process. A plant-based diet contains antioxidants, which neutralize damaging free radicals and prevent normal cells from aging prematurely or mutating.

All these benefits have evolved in plants over thousands of years to protect them from disease, the sun, and the elements. Now they can protect you. Eat abundantly from plant foods and you will build up a shield of internal body armor few cancer cells can pierce.

DIABETES

Diabetes is ravaging the world at an astonishing rate. One in eleven Americans suffers from the disease; nearly four thousand new cases hit the streets every day, and researchers suspect that as many as one in three people born after 2000 will develop it sometime in their lives. To put it bluntly, diabetes will soon transition from being an epidemic to a pandemic.

Diabetes is the leading cause of blindness, amputation, and kidney failure. Diabetes doubles your chance of having a heart attack or stroke. Diabetes wreaks havoc on your vascular system, turning once-healthy blood vessels sickly.

The economic toll of this epidemic is severe. In 2012, for example, the annual cost of diabetes in America was $245 billion—that's roughly equivalent to one out of every 5 health care dollars spent in this country.

There are two different types of diabetes—Type 1, which accounts for 5 to 10 percent of all cases and usually appears at an early age, and Type 2, which accounts for the remaining cases. They are very different animals.

In Type 1 diabetes, the pancreas can no longer produce insulin, the hormone necessary for getting sugar, or glucose, into your cells to provide your body with the energy they need to work. Imagine that every cell has a door with a lock. Insulin is the key that fits into the lock, turns, and swings open the door to deliver the glucose.

Researchers now believe one way pancreatic insulin cells get wiped out in Type 1 diabetes is through friendly fire—i.e., an immune system reaction.

That fire can come from something as seemingly innocent as cow's milk. For example, an infant's immature digestive tract can't always completely digest milk protein. This undigested protein, which slips through the semipermeable membrane of the small intestine into the bloodstream, appears to the immune system to be a foreign invader. The baby's body responds by attacking the undigested protein like a pack of great white sharks.

While on the attack, the immune system seeks out other invaders that might be lurking, and mistakenly attacks the infant's pancreatic insulin-producing cells, which resemble the protein in cow's milk. The great white sharks of the immune system then tear to shreds and gobble up the baby's pancreatic insulin-producing cells. The victim is now a Type 1 diabetic for life.

IN TYPE 2 DIABETES, the pancreas still produces insulin, but it is no longer effective in getting glucose into the cells.

When you consume a high-fat, animal-based diet, your body's cells start to gunk up and cake over with fat. It's okay for them to contain some fat as a backup energy source, but beyond a certain level, your insulin "key" can no longer open the cell doors because it, too, is all gummed up with fat and debris. The glucose you need now ends up circulating in your bloodstream. You are now what's called insulin-resistant, and well on your way to becoming a Type 2 diabetic.

(This type of diabetes used to be called adult-onset diabetes, as it affected only adults. However, with Americans becoming unhealthy and obese at an increasingly younger age, so many kids have been coming down with diabetes that the medical profession had to rename the disease.)

BACK AT THE STATION, we were making more and more diabetic-related calls. Here's one:

After piling into the fire engine and driving to the scene of the alarm, we arrived to find a car in a ditch, smashed into a telephone pole. The driver of the car, a man in his early fifties, wore a glazed expression and, based on looking at him through the car windows, seemed completely out of it. All the car doors were locked, and the man kept shifting back and forth, not knowing what to do.

We repeatedly asked him to open the door so we could help him. He didn't respond.

Then we noticed he was wearing a diabetic emergency bracelet, and we put two and two together. His blood sugar must have sunk too low and caused him to lose control of his car and drive into the pole. We again asked him to talk to us.

However, he kept looking at us with a blank stare as if we were speaking ancient Greek.

After realizing that we weren't going to be able to communicate with the man, we took out Mr. Pinky (a thick, pink coat hanger–type contraption that allows us to access locked cars), opened the driver's door, and began patient care.

The man's blood sugar turned out to be 32 mg/dl, which is far too low for anyone to function. So we fed him two 15-gram tubes of glucose, and within five minutes he came out of his zombie-like state and was back on planet Earth. He apologized profusely, saying he must not have eaten enough at lunch. We backed him out of the ditch and told him that he needed to get some solid food into his system as soon as possible.

THE TRUTH IS THAT TREATING TYPE 2 DIABETES is an easy fix. Eat plant-strong!

Neal Barnard, MD, is president of the Physicians Committee for Responsible Medicine, and author of *Dr. Neal Barnard's Program for Reversing Diabetes*. The results of his diabetes studies, funded by the National Institutes of Health, were published in the August 2006 issue of *Diabetes Care*.

In his report, Dr. Barnard describes a simple dietary regime he found that could prevent, control, and even reverse diabetes. Of the ninety-nine patients in his study, fifty were put on the American Diabetes Association (ADA) diet (currently considered the nutritional gold standard for people with diabetes). The other forty-nine subjects ate a low-fat, high-fiber, plant-based diet.

In choosing which foods to eat in which quantities, the ADA diet patients followed the standard USDA food pyramid, but also had to count calories and watch portion sizes. No food group was eliminated, however. The plant-based diet patients followed the Physicians Committee food pyramid, which features more servings of whole grains, vegetables, fruits, and legumes than the standard pyramid. These patients could eat as much as they wanted as long as they ate only from these four food groups and watched their intake of nuts and high-fat vegetables such as olives and avocados.

The group of diabetics on the low-fat, plant-based diet was able to reduce the doses of almost all their medications, and in some cases go off them, in as few as twelve weeks. This diet also turned out to be three times more effective than the ADA diet in reducing A1C, a marker that best identifies the amount of sugar in the blood over a three-month period.

Why was Dr. Barnard's study so successful? The answer is so simple, it's criminal: Because eating low-fat, plant-scrumptious foods causes the body to burn and metabolize excess fat from all the cells of the body. So in as little as a week, insulin can knock on the cell door, stick its golden key in the now-clean lock, and turn it. The door is now open and insulin can deliver its glucose. Once that happens, a person is no longer insulin-resistant, but insulin-sensitive.

Several E2ers have been able to reverse their Type 2 diabetes. For example, Craig Walker, a twenty-four-year veteran of the fire department, had been diagnosed with Type 2 diabetes at age forty-one. Six years later he came to me after hearing about the success I'd had in improving the health of some of the other firefighters. "I'm finally ready to try this," he said. "I am sick and tired of being sick and tired."

Coming out of the fire academy, fire cadet Craig weighed 185 pounds and was healthy as a moose (yes, a moose, as my childhood pediatrician used to tell me at the end of a checkup). More than two decades later, Captain Craig Walker weighed 215 pounds, had a high A1C of 12, and a fasting blood sugar level of over 200, gave himself an insulin shot daily, took two oral diabetic medications, and had just quit Lipitor for high cholesterol because he didn't like the way it made him feel.

By going on the E2 diet, in just three months Craig lost 27 pounds, brought his A1C number down from 12 to 6.5, brought his fasting glucose level below 100, no longer needed his insulin injections, was able to stop taking one oral medication and cut the other dose in half, reduced his total cholesterol from 269 to 196, and cut his LDL cholesterol from 189 to 111.

Craig is no longer sick and tired. Craig is healthy and happy—as a moose!

Carol Jocelyn, 66
Director of a House of Prayer

I live in rural Iowa, one of the beef- and pork-eating capitals of America, so some people think I'm nuts. But the nice thing is that even people who live in remote places like me can make it work if they want. I travel to health food stores whenever I'm away. And I'm helping to integrate more healthy foods into our regular grocery store. Today my energy is at a wonderful peak, my body feels clean, I feel alive, and I've lost eighteen pounds. I've gone from a size twelve to a size eight.

OBESITY

Our country is in terrible shape—physically, that is. We are fat. Dr. Richard Carmona, the former United States surgeon general, refers to the nation's current obesity epidemic as "the terror within."

If you are obese (like more than 30 percent of all Americans), you're essentially stepping onto an escalator taking you directly into a roomful of killer diseases: heart disease, stroke, cancer, hypertension, and diabetes. Once inside this room, you'll realize the absolute horror that lies within, but the door will close and won't let you leave until you pick one or more diseases as a departing prize.

On every shift at the station we saw the results of the obesity epidemic in full swing. Sometimes we get a call for what's known as lifting assistance; this type of help is for people so morbidly obese that they have lost their mobility. Lifting and moving people who weigh between four hundred and six hundred pounds requires a team effort, as well as a great deal of resourcefulness.

First, we gather the required man/woman power (usually six to eight people) and two bedsheets. Next, we help the person roll onto his or her side, and slide the two sheets up against the body. Then we have the person roll back onto his or her back and then to the other side so we can pull the sheet past and under, giving us a makeshift gurney.

Now comes the exciting part: Positioned all around the sheet, each person rolls up his or her section to get a solid grip. On the count of three, we then slide the patient over to one side of the bed and prepare to lift him or her onto the stretcher or straight into an ambulance. Considering that we often have to navigate our way around furniture, through doorways, and down multiple staircases, this task can be pretty difficult.

AMERICANS SEEM TO FEEL it is their birthright to eat rich, fatty, meaty, and obesity-promoting foods. This mind-set begs for a paradigm shift. Obesity is not caused by a fat gene passed down the family line; its roots lie in bad eating habits and poor nutrition. These habits are the colossal tragedy being passed from one generation to the next.

There is a solution, and it doesn't involve portion control, exercise, or lifting weights. It requires one thing and one thing only: You need to become plant-strong! Indulge in the luxuriance of eating plants and discover the wide variety of foods that await you.

Here are some basic truths about gaining (far too much) weight.

First, you will gain weight only if you consume more calories than you burn. Stop eating high-calorie second- and third-class foods such as meat, cheese, milk, eggs, oils, and refined sugars and replace them with first-class, opulent, plant-based foods, then watch the pounds disappear.

Second, people around the world whose diets are plant-based tend to be thinner than those whose aren't. Their cuisine is rich in complex carbohydrates such as whole grains, potatoes, millet, rice, and corn, and they supplement these healthful starches with fruits, vegetables, and beans. It works for them, and it will work for you.

TO UNDERSTAND WHY THIS IS THE CASE, here's a quick lesson on how calories work, and the basics of how the body processes the three types of macronutrients found in all foods: protein, carbohydrates, and fats.

A gram of each contains a different number of calories:

1 gram of carbohydrate equals 4 calories.
1 gram of protein equals 4 calories.
1 gram of fat equals 9 calories.

Carbohydrates, the body's main source of fuel, are stored in the form of glucose in the blood and glycogen in the muscles and liver. Just in the process of converting and storing these carbs, the body burns off 25 percent of the calories you consume.

The body cannot store protein, however. Excess protein is either eliminated in the feces or urine, or stored as fat. If protein were stored as muscle, 90 percent of Americans would be walking around resembling body-building champions. Look around, and you will quickly see that this is far from the case.

Meanwhile, the human body requires only a minuscule percentage of its daily calories from fat—roughly 3 to 5 percent. Yet most Americans are choking down upward of 40 percent of their daily calories in the form of fat, a large portion of which is unhealthy saturated fat.

The body has evolved to store extra fat in a very efficient manner. Only a measly 2 percent of fat calories are burned up when fat is stored.

This is why the fat you eat is the fat you wear, as Dr. John McDougall has said.

Most animal-based foods contain between 20 and 60 percent fat, whereas most plant-based foods contain less than 10 percent fat. And animal products contain no fiber, while the naturally occurring fiber in plant-based foods allows you to become full without having to pile in so many calories.

There is nothing in an animal-product-based diet that you cannot find in a healthier, safer, and better form in a plant-based diet.

Why? Because plant foods contain all of the essential amino acids found in protein, both of the essential fatty acids (linoleic and alpha-linolenic), all of the thirteen vitamins, and all of the seven major and nine minor minerals. And they can supply these nourishing macro- and micronutrients without subjecting you to any of the toxic side effects of animal products— namely, premature disease and death.

As previously discussed, the only vitamin plants don't provide is vitamin B12. The microorganisms in the soil that once supplied our diets with B12 naturally have been stripped away by current farming methods, so plant eaters must add this vitamin to their diet.

The current recommendation is for 500 micrograms per day, but if you consume milk substitutes and cereals, you are already eating products fortified with B12 and are more than likely getting enough. If not, consider taking a supplement.

LET ME REPEAT: THE ANSWER to putting out a fire is water. The answer to stamping out obesity is a plant-based diet. We all need to grab buckets of plant-based foods and work as a team to douse the obesity crisis.

Losing weight is not rocket science and it's not magic. It's just the simple law of eating only constructive foods and omitting destructive ones. With the Engine 2 Diet, you'll need only four weeks to lay a foundation that can last a lifetime.

ALZHEIMER'S DISEASE/DEMENTIA

Alzheimer's disease and dementia currently affect forty-four million people worldwide, and are predicted to increase fivefold by 2050. They affect one in nine Americans older than sixty-five, and close to 33 percent of people older than eighty.

The two diseases present themselves in similar ways, but the mechanisms that create them differ.

Dementia (cognitive impairment) is the result of many tiny strokes called TIAs, which we talked about earlier. They're also called silent strokes because victims rarely realize anything has happened to them. After a TIA, you typically suffer a mild level of mental impairment lasting an hour or two, and then return to normal. TIAs often occur while you are sleeping, eating, or going about normal activities.

The human brain rebounds quickly because it has such an amazing reserve capacity. It isn't until we've had multiple TIAs that our brain starts losing the battle, and a swift downward slide to mental oblivion follows.

Alzheimer's disease, on the other hand, seems to result from plaque formation. However, instead of sticking to the artery walls leading to your heart, brain, pelvis, or legs, these plaques develop in the pockets between your brain cells.

Such plaques are composed of a rogue protein called beta-amyloid. Numerous studies have shown a direct correlation between the amount of cholesterol and fat in the diet and the amount of beta-amyloid protein buildup in the body.

I once traveled to Austin's Station 9 to fill in for another firefighter who was out sick. Over the course of my twenty-four-hour shift, I had a heartfelt conversation with a firefighter friend and fellow triathlete named Patrick. Patrick's father had suffered a heart attack and respiratory arrest at age sixty-two and had started losing his mind to dementia at age seventy; two years later, Patrick and his mother moved him into a nursing home. The man's perceptions of reality changed like a kaleidoscope; one minute he'd think he was in the Vietnam War, the next he'd be in his hometown of Copperas Cove, Texas.

Patrick told me that the saddest moment in his life was when he looked into his father's eyes and realized his dad had no idea who Patrick was. Patrick then told me not only that his father had been a smoker all his life, but that he had eaten anything and everything that came his way.

Patrick feared that he might be prone to the same fate as his father. I told him that that was not the case; plenty of research exists showing that you can lower your risk of Alzheimer's. In fact, a 2003 report in the *Annual Review of Public Health* stressed that lifestyle and diet play a major role in the development of this disease, and that it's never too late to take action—especially if you have a family history that puts you at increased risk in the first place.

Other studies also point in this direction. For example, researchers at the Ninth International Conference on Alzheimer's Disease and Related Disorders reported in 2004 that obesity, high cholesterol, and high blood pressure significantly heighten the risk of Alzheimer's. The researchers followed a group of 1,500 older subjects for twenty-one years and found a combination of all three factors increased that risk sixfold.

The same study, released in the 2005 issue of *The Lancet Neurology,* reported that older people who exercised at least twice a week had a roughly 60 percent lower risk of suffering from Alzheimer's and dementia than their couch potato peers. The theory is that exercise helps ward off Alzheimer's by boosting blood flow to the brain and protecting its blood vessels.

Meanwhile, a four-year study of 815 Chicago seniors (reported in the February 2003 issue of the *Archives of Neurology*) found that a diet high in saturated fat doubles the risk of developing Alzheimer's.

Myriad other studies have linked Alzheimer's with high levels of a substance called homocysteine. Homocysteine is an amino acid, one of the building blocks of proteins. It is created by the liver when we consume another essential amino acid called methionine. The quantity of methionine found in animal protein is two to three times greater than in plant protein, so it follows that eating meat and dairy can easily raise your homocysteine levels to a dangerous degree.

Another study from the July 2000 World Alzheimer Congress had more promising news. Researchers examined 5,395 individuals aged fifty-five and older who were free from dementia in 1993, and again in 1999. The results: "On average, people who remained free from any form of dementia had consumed higher amounts of beta-carotene, vitamin C, vitamin E and vegetables than the people in the study who developed Alzheimer's disease."

The researchers also noted that two risk factors for Alzheimer's, family history and a genetic marker, did not alter their findings. High consumption of vegetables appeared to offset the other known risk factors for Alzheimer's.

Don't take your mind for granted. Since a major risk factor for Alzheimer's is associated with an animal-based diet, while reduced risk is associated with a plant-based diet, why not give your mind a break and give up the steak?

Linda Liebowitz, 48
Housewife

It's not just my cholesterol level (from 266 to 167) and my weight that have dropped so much (I went from a size ten to a size six)—my grocery bill has dropped, too. When you've got a family of four, that's all the reward you need.

I HOPE IT IS NOW CRYSTAL CLEAR to you how many of us are suffering from the foods at the end of our forks. It is nothing short of a travesty. Here we are, living in the great land of America in the twenty-first century, possessing the knowledge to fight off our most crippling diseases, yet we continue to consume excess amounts of toxic animal protein, fat, and cholesterol, as well as processed and refined foods.

Medical science has shown us that the American diet is unhealthy. Yet modern medicine still treats all these diseases without addressing their root cause: improper nutrition.

For example, doctors address our worst epidemic, cardiovascular disease, by treating only the symptoms. They are attempting to solve a molecular problem with mechanical tools. And these tools, such as cholesterol-lowering drugs and fancy surgeries using all kinds of gadgets from wire cages to balloons, do not extend life and don't prevent new heart attacks.

We firefighters are part of the problem, too. Despite our emphasis on safety, rescue, and fitness, the career with the greatest incidence of heart attacks is, indeed, firefighting. Trust me, if you were a fly on the wall at a firehouse, you would be amazed to watch what the majority of firefighters eat!

EXTINGUISHING FIRE AND DISEASE

Firefighters want to, and do, save lives. Occasionally our jobs require us to rush into a burning building and pull out victims. That's a drastic measure. We'd prefer to teach people how to prevent a fire from ever occurring in the first place.

Bad health is like a raging fire in the body, and can be just as deadly. The best way to fireproof yourself is to eat a whole grain, plant-strong diet.

The chances of starting a fire and/or promoting disease are greatly reduced if you follow these rules in each area.

FIRE PREVENTION

1. Working smoke detectors save lives. They're like big noses that sniff for smoke and never go to sleep. But as we like to say in the Austin Fire Department, "Put a finger on it" once a month to make sure the batteries work. And change them twice yearly.

2. Keep a fire extinguisher in the kitchen. Kitchen fires account for the majority of house fires. Don't get distracted and leave cooking food unattended.

3. Candles are fire candy. Use them only when someone is in the room, and make sure they're in a secure holder, away from combustible materials.

4. Matches and lighters are tools, not toys. Teach your children that they are for adults only.

5. Plan your escape in case of fire. Know at least two ways out of every room. Create a designated meeting place outside your home. Tell children never to hide under a bed, in a closet, or in a bathtub.

6. Crawl low under smoke. Our saying in Austin is: "Get low and go." Clean air is always nearest the floor. Drop and head immediately to one of your two exits.

7. If your clothes catch fire, don't run. Stop, drop, and roll. Stop where you are, drop to the ground, cover your face with your hands, and roll over and over to smother the flames.

8. Don't smoke. Smoldering cigarette butts cause fires and are the number one cause of fire death in the United States. If you're a smoker, for heaven's sake, don't fall asleep smoking on the couch or in bed, because heaven's where you'll end up.

DISEASE PREVENTION

1. Eat green leafy vegetables like there is no tomorrow: broccoli, bok choy, mustard greens, kale, collard greens, spinach, romaine lettuce, and Brussels sprouts. No other foods are as nutrient dense.

2. Eat plant foods of all the colors of the rainbow every day: red, green, blue, yellow, orange, and purple. Maximize the massive variety of phytochemicals and antioxidants by consuming these nutrient-rich food bombs. Watch your palate and energy change before your eyes.

3. Fiber is your friend. Eat fruits, vegetables, whole grains, and beans and you'll get all the fiber you'll ever need. You'll consistently feel better and your bowels will be as regular as clockwork.

4. Get junk food out of the house. If it's in the cupboard, you'll be drawn to it like a moth to light. Don't torture yourself. Toss it!

5. Always carry food with you: whole grain crackers, healthy energy bars, fruit, or vegetables. Don't let a hungry stomach lead you astray.

6. If you smoke, stop. And if you don't smoke, don't start. It isn't cool, smart, or worth it.

7. Minimize or eliminate the booze. It's not healthy and rarely enhances life.

8. Get off your butt and move. No matter how good your diet is, you need to exercise your body. Do anything as long as your heart thumps and your blood pumps. Life is better after a workout.

6

THE E2
EXERCISE PROGRAM

Fighting a fire is more demanding than running a triathlon. It requires a combination of strength, endurance, stamina, and mental acuity; you have to be firing on all cylinders to perform the tough tasks that can be required of you at any minute during your twenty-four-hour shift.

Every time the alarm goes off, the following hour could be the most challenging of your life. And that alarm doesn't care if you're in the middle of dinner, shampooing your hair, or dead asleep. You have to respond.

Several years ago Engine 2 responded to a high-rise fire. Such a situation requires firefighters to deal with both high population density and a huge fire load—a recipe for potential disaster.

The fire turned out to be on the twenty-third floor of one of the city's tallest buildings. Although the elevators automatically shut down in such cases, firefighters have a special key to operate them. In this case, however, the key didn't work, so we had to take the stairs.

Climbing twenty-three flights is never easy, but imagine doing it hauling 100 pounds of supplies. There's your bunker gear, which weighs about 20 pounds; an air pack, which weighs 35 pounds; and a high-rise hose, which weighs around 50 pounds. Then there are the tools and flashlights, and someone also has to hoist the high-rise pack, which contains wrenches and other gear.

This is what I had to endure with my buddies from Engine 1: Russ, Josh, Wayne, and JR. By the time we got to the tenth floor, two of them were gasping for air; they could barely walk. So the remaining three of us took the high-rise hose and pack and climbed the remaining thirteen flights of stairs.

Luckily, the fire didn't turn out to be serious—it was just some smoke from a burned-out elevator motor—but imagine how the others would have felt if something tragic had happened on the twenty-third floor.

These sorts of physical demands are another reason the firefighters at Engine 2 took up the plant-strong diet plan with a vengeance. In fact, physical exercise is a great adjunct to the Engine 2 Diet because, when taken together, you'll see your weight, and your cholesterol level, drop even lower than you ever imagined!

There are two components to getting yourself into adequate Engine 2–quality physical shape. The first is exercising the *cardiovascular system* (the heart and lungs), which is worked whenever you do anything aerobic in nature. You should try to get cardiovascular exercise, which elevates the heart rate, gets the blood pumping, tones muscles, and burns calories, twenty to forty minutes a day. This can be achieved by an aggressive walk or by jogging, running, biking, swimming, rowing, or cross-country skiing.

The second is exercising the *muscular system*, worked whenever you do some form of strength or resistance training.

The beauty of the Engine 2 strength training program is that each round of exercises works both the cardiovascular system as well as the muscular system.

My recommendation is that you aim to exercise at least five days a week, whether cardiovascular or strength training, for anywhere from ten to forty-five minutes. Ten minutes? Yes, even ten minutes counts! If you're busy and ten minutes is all you've got, use it. Oh, ya! Those ten short minutes will do wonders. On many days the twenty-minute bike ride from my house to Whole Foods Global is the only exercise I get—yet it makes me feel so invigorated, I'm on top of my game.

Fun fact: The longest word in the English language with one vowel happens to be *strengths*. But for most people, this is where the fun ends, as the thought of strength training conjures up images of weights and barbells, muscle heads and gyms, and lots of time and too much money.

There is a better way. It's called *Engine 2 Strength Training.* By relying on your own body weight instead of metal weights, you can avoid the crowds at the gym, instead exercising in the comfort of a park or your own home, maximizing your time and energy, and do it all for zero money.

Why is strength/resistance training so important? First, added strength will allow you to perform better in life—a life that requires you to stand, lunge, bend, twist, and lift on a daily basis.

Second, you will be strengthening not only your muscles, but also your bones. Dropping all animal protein from your diet in conjunction with strength training is a must for preventing osteoporosis.

Third, as we age, our muscles atrophy at an accelerated rate in a process called sarcopenia. This weakening can be prevented and even reversed with consistent strength training.

Finally, by consuming a calorie-light and nutrient-heavy plant-powered diet, complemented with a strength training program, you will give your body a beautiful one-two combination punch that will maximize weight loss in the healthiest and most effective manner.

Keep up the exercise and you'll even burn calories while you're *not* working out! By replacing your body's slow-burning fat with fast-burning muscle, you will be increasing your RMR (resting metabolic rate). This is the rate at which your body burns calories while you are resting, sitting, and even sleeping. When you replace fat with muscle, you'll increase your RMR many times over.

In addition to increasing weight loss and ramping up your RMR, strength training will also provide your physique with firmness and muscle tone. You'll look magnificent!

Audrey Cravotta, 16
Student

Sometimes I hear weird things from other kids, like, "Dude, your hair's going to start falling out." But then I also get things like, "Hey, your skin looks really great," and that makes up for it. Because that's true. Also, I've lost ten pounds—and actually, my hair's never been healthier.

BEFORE GETTING STARTED

Looking back over my life, I can't remember ever going more than two days in a row without engaging in some type of exercise. Exercise has become as much a part of my life as brushing my teeth and eating plant-based food—it's my cup of coffee in the morning; it's my nightcap in the evening. If I can't fit in at least ten minutes of exercise a day, I don't feel centered. And when I do get my exercise, I feel wonderful.

Most of you probably don't feel the same way—yet. But as these exercises help tone and strengthen, they'll flood your body with endorphins, your brain's happy-making chemicals.

While some of you may never have attempted anything like this before, and may struggle a bit, other readers may be fit as a triathlete. So I've designed the following circuit training for all ability levels—I've put everyone from overweight moms and dads to professional athletes through this program.

Please be sure to consult your doctor before beginning any exercise program. Then, start where you're comfortable, and as your strength, coordination, agility, and confidence improve, move up a level. Stay consistent and stay committed and your body will respond swiftly. As you progress, know that someone out there is very, very proud of you (me).

BEFORE STARTING THE E2 EXERCISES, I suggest warming up with a set of Carl Sandburg stretches, invented by the great American poet of the same name, who did them every morning until the age of ninety-three. His daughter Helga Sandburg (whom my grandfather, Dr. Barney Crile, married after his first wife died) still performed these exercises every morning herself until she passed away in 2014 at the age of ninety-five.

Here are six of the best Sandburg stretches for you to do every day. These will wake up your nervous system, boost your heart rate and core temperature, and increase your muscular elasticity. (To see all the Sandburg stretches, go to www.engine2diet.com.)

The Carl Sandburg Stretches

1. Sun Salutations

Start in the standing position with your hands by your sides, then bend over and touch your toes (or as far as you can reach). Now, very slowly stretch your hands up toward the sky, letting your back bend slightly. Repeat this ten times.

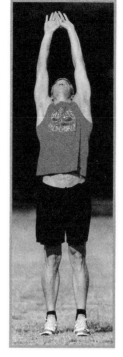
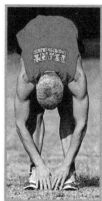

2. Kicking Toe Touches

Start with your right arm and hand straight out in front of your body, then kick up your left leg, trying to come as close as possible to touch your hand. Now, do the reverse: Raise your left arm and hand, then kick up your right foot to meet your left hand. Do this move ten times, alternating from side to side.

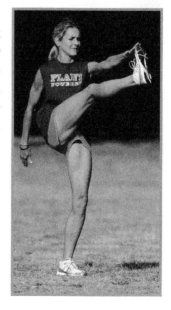

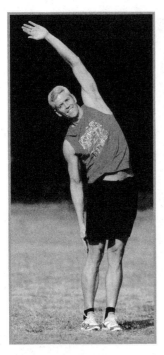

3. Side Stretches

Start with your left arm straight up in the air, leaving your right arm hanging by your side. Move your right hand down toward your right calf, letting your left arm move over your head (your body will curve to the right). Then, repeat this move to the opposite side, raising the right arm and stretching to the left. Perform this motion ten times in each direction.

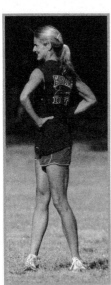

4. Trunk Twists

Start with your hands on your hips. Twist your torso to the left, then to the right. Do ten stretches to each side.

5. Barrel Rolls

Start with your hands on your hips. Now, bend your torso to the right. Then, in one flowing motion, move it forward to the left, and finally back to your starting position. Now repeat the roll but reverse your direction. Roll in each direction (right to left, then left to right) ten times.

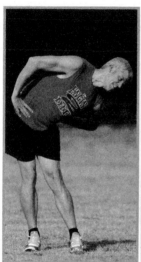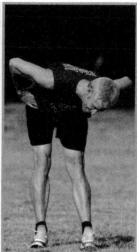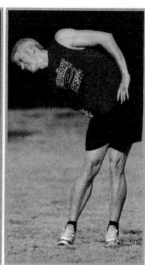

6. Arm Circles

Start by holding your arms straight out by your side, perpendicular to your body. Now move both arms using a circular motion, tracing rings in the air. Do ten forward circles, then ten backward circles.

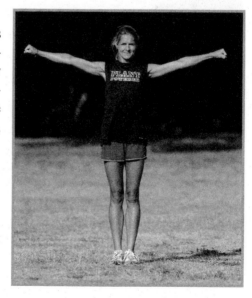

THE E2 EXERCISE PROGRAM

I recommend doing the following Engine 2 Exercise Program twice a week. This will serve you well as a strength training and aerobic workout. The shorter the rest interval you take between each exercise, the better aerobic workout you will receive. In addition, another three times during the week enjoy a pure aerobic activity for twenty to forty minutes. This can include walking, jogging, biking, swimming, rowing, basketball, and/or tennis. The goal is to get the heart rate elevated to about 70 to 80 percent of maximum.

Here is a chart to help you schedule each during the twenty-eight days.

The ENGINE 2 DIET

	EASY EXERCISE PLANNER			
▼ ▼ ▼ ▼ ▼ ▼ ▼	WEEK 1	WEEK 2	WEEK 3	WEEK 4
DAY 1	E2 Strength		Aerobic	
DAY 2		E2 Strength		E2 Strength
DAY 3	Aerobic	Aerobic	E2 Strength	Serobic
DAY 4	Aerobic	Aerobic	Aerobic	Aerobic
DAY 5				
DAY 6	E2 Strength	E2 Strength	Aerobic	E2 Strength
DAY 7	Aerobic	Aerobic	E2 Strength	Aerobic

The E2 Exercise Program consists of three rounds of four exercises. All three rounds combine simple body strength exercises along with an aerobic exercise.

Each round follows this rhythm: First you work the large, powerful leg muscles. Second, you work the upper body muscles of the chest, back, shoulders, and arms. Third, you focus on the supporting muscles surrounding the spine and hip area, known as the core. Each round ends with a cardiovascular exercise to target the heart and lungs.

Round 1

1. Legs: Body Weight Air Squats

These little puppies don't seem like much at first, but once you get up to 50-plus repetitions, they rock'n'roll.

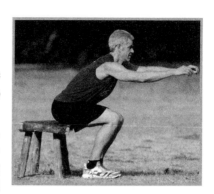

Standing in front of a chair, bench, or Swiss ball with your feet shoulder-width apart, pretend you are going to sit down, lowering your bottom until it barely touches the surface. Then rise back up to the standing position.

Form is important. Sit back into the squat with your heels, not your toes.

Beginners: 10 to 15 reps.

Intermediate: 20 to 40 reps.

Advanced: 75 to 100 reps.

2. Upper Body: Push-Ups

The standard push-up is a wonderful, time-honored body weight exercise for everyone. Begin by assuming the plank position, or the starting position for all push-ups: Lie down on your stomach, place your toes and hands on the ground, then push up on your arms so your back is straight, not swayed—as if there were a plank between your head and feet. Next, lower yourself down toward the ground, stopping when your nose and chest are one inch away. Remember to keep your abs slightly engaged. Now push yourself up to the starting plank position again.

Beginners: Do incline push-ups. Here, instead of lying on the ground, brace yourself against a wall, table, countertop, or desk—at any angle you can handle. Lower yourself on a three count, hold it for one count, and then push up on a three count. Do 10 reps.

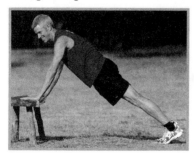 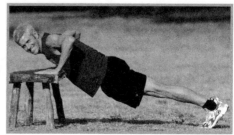

Intermediate: Do 25 reps of normal push-ups. If you start to fizzle out, lower your knees to the ground, take a small break, and finish the set.

Advanced: Do normal push-ups, but with your right leg, then your left leg, raised in the air for 10 reps each. Next, place both feet down for a final 20 reps, for 40 reps total.

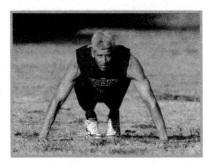 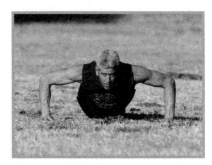

3. Core: Flutter Kicks

This is a fun exercise. Pretend you just fell off the *Titanic* and your only hope of survival depends on your being able to kick your way over to a lifeboat one hundred yards away (you will make it, by the way!). Lie down on your back with your hands under your tailbone. Raise your legs together 6 to 12 inches off the floor. Now move one leg up and one leg down in a deliberate, scissors-type motion. Each kick counts as one repetition. (Concentrate on keeping your lower back pressed down into the floor to avoid straining your back.)

Beginners: 20 reps.

Intermediate: 100 reps.

Advanced: 200 reps.

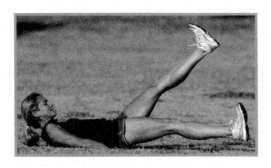

4. Cardiovascular: Squat Thrusts or Burbies

This exercise works the heart and lungs as well as developing your agility, timing, coordination, and strength. Begin in the standing position with your hands by your sides. Now bend over and place your hands on the ground 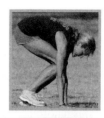 in front of each foot. Keep your legs slightly bent. Next, throw both legs behind you like a kicking donkey so you are in the plank pose. Immediately bring both legs back up to your chest so you are once again in the squatting position. Last, stand back up.

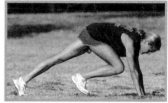

Beginners: Walk your legs back one at a time into the plank position instead of thrusting them, then walk back into the squatting position, then stand up: 10 reps.

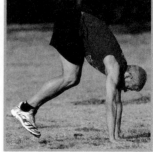

Intermediate: Squat down, donkey-kick your legs out into the plank position, thrust them back in to your chest, and then instead of standing up, jump in the air: 20 reps.

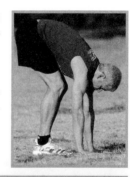

Advanced: After thrusting your legs out into the plank position, add a push-up, then thrust your legs back to your chest and stand: 30 reps.

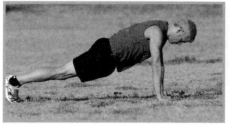

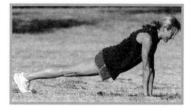

Round 2

1. Legs: Lunges

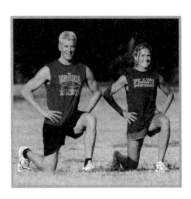

The standard lunge is a graceful and dynamic exercise, and a must for anyone who wants to build leg strength, improve balance, and get chiseled muscles.

Start by standing upright with your feet shoulder-width apart. Take a large step forward with your right leg and lower yourself until your thigh is parallel with the floor or your opposite knee gently hits the ground. Next, push backward off the same leg and return to the starting position. Repeat with the left leg. This completes one lunge repetition.

(Be sure to keep your hands by your side or on your hips for balance and stability; don't rest them on your thighs.)

Beginners: 5 reps.

Intermediate: 10 reps.

Advanced: 20 reps, and holding 5- to 10-pound weights in each hand. (The weights may be in the form of canned goods, heavy pieces of fruit, or even the blocks of cheese and meat you'll be throwing out.)

2. Upper Body: Seated Chair Dips

This exercise feels like a breeze at first, and then about three-quarters of the way through, it starts to burn—but so very nicely.

Sit in a chair or on a bench, then slide yourself forward so your bottom starts to fall off the front. Grasp the front of the chair or bench with your palms placed downward and your fingers pointed forward. Keep your feet pointed upward so your weight is on your heels and not your toes. Lower yourself with a straight back until your arms are at a 90-degree angle. Now push yourself back to the starting position.

Beginners: Keep your knees bent at 90 degrees, with the soles of your feet on the ground, going down until your arms are parallel with the chair: 5 to 10 reps.

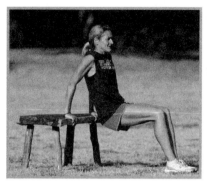
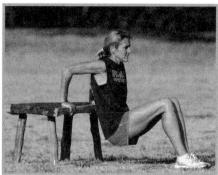

Intermediate: Place your legs straight out in front of you with heels on the ground: 30 to 50 reps.

Advanced: Use the same form as intermediate, but do 60 to 80 reps.

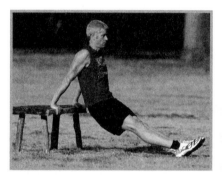
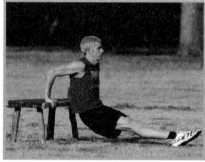

3. Core: Plank Pose

This core exercise works the abs, the pelvic floor, the hips, and the stabilizing muscles of the back. Get ready for a sweet burn and, perhaps, to shake like a leaf.

When doing this exercise, remember to engage your abs and extend out through your head and through your feet. I challenge you to work up to 5 minutes of this—if you can, you are an Engine 2 workout animal!

To do the plank pose, lie facedown and place your toes and elbows on the ground. Then push up so your back is perfectly straight.

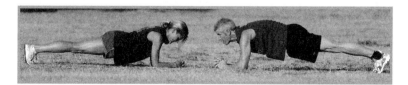

Beginners: 30 seconds. Stay in this pose for as long as possible, but use your knees if necessary (take as many 5-second breaks as you need until you can work up to 30 seconds).

Intermediate: Stay 2 minutes (take 2-second breaks if necessary).

Advanced: Hold on for 5 minutes (or at least 4)!

4. Cardiovascular: Jumping Jacks

This is an old-time favorite that you probably did in middle or high school gym class. It is an excellent cardio exercise, especially when performed very fast.

Start in a standing position with your hands by your sides. Jump up while spreading your legs apart and touching your hands together over your head. After you land, jump up again, this time bringing your legs back together and your arms by your sides. The move counts as one jumping jack.

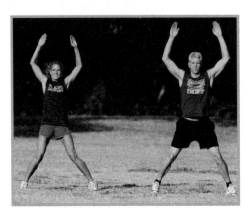

Beginners: 20 reps.

Intermediate: 50 reps.

Advanced: 100 reps.

(For the really advanced, try Funky Feet Jumping Jacks: Do a regular jumping jack, followed by one in which you place your right foot forward and left foot back, then another placing your left foot forward and right foot back. Finally, do another regular jumping jack.)

Round 3

1. Legs: Step-Ups

I loved doing this exercise when I trained for triathlons. I'd run a quarter mile, do ten step-ups with each leg, and then run another quarter mile. It was a nice simulation of how it felt to run after working out my legs on the bike. I now incorporate step-ups into my exercise routine to aid in developing my leg strength, for when I have to climb stairs carrying my sleeping kids.

Find a step or a bench that is level with or stands just below your knee. Place one foot flat on top of the step and then push into a standing position. Lower yourself in a smooth, controlled motion.

Note: This exercise's effectiveness is dependent on pushing off with your raised leg and keeping the rear leg completely relaxed.

As your strength improves, you can increase the height of the step and/or hold some weights in your hands (soup cans or 5-pound dumbbells).

Beginners: Use your body weight only, doing 5 to 10 reps on each leg.

Intermediate: Add 5-pound weights in each hand. Do 15 to 25 reps on each leg.

Advanced: Add 10 pounds in each hand; do 30 reps on each leg.

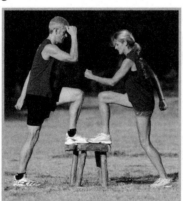
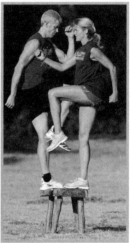

2. Upper Body: Downward Dogs

Namaste! It's time to tap into your inner yogi. I've been doing yoga for more than twenty years and absolutely love it. It is a centering and relaxing workout.

The downward dog is a combination strength and stretch move and should be a mainstay in everyone's yoga repertoire. To do it, make your body an inverted V by placing your weight on your hands and feet and holding your bottom high in the air. Concentrate on breathing in through your nose—letting the breath fill up your belly and then exhaling slow and steady on a three count.

Beginners: Hold the downward dog position for 5 slow and relaxing breaths followed immediately by 15 to 30 seconds of child's pose. Get on your knees and sit back so your bottom is resting on the soles of your feet, then lean forward with your arms over your head and place your forehead on the ground and completely surrender yourself to gravity. Do 3 to 5 rounds.

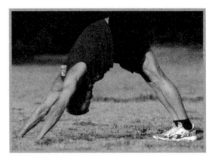

Intermediate: Downward dog for 5 slow and relaxed breaths followed by 5 push-ups. Do 5 rounds.

Advanced: Downward dog for 5 slow and relaxed breaths followed by 10 push-ups. Do 5 rounds!

3. Core: V-Ups or Pike-Ups

These exercises can help you get the proverbial six pack—or at least, so claim people who do them.

Depending on your ability, do one of two exercises: seated V-ups or pike-ups.

Seated V-up: Sit on your butt with your arms by your sides, your hands on the ground and your fingers pointed forward, and your feet flat on the ground. Pull your knees together into your chest, raise your feet off the ground two to three inches, and balance on your butt. Extend your legs and feet forward on a five count until they are straight out in front of you. Hold this pose for one second and then bring your knees back to your chest.

Pike-up: I learned this exercise from watching the University of Texas diving team as I swam up and down the adjacent pool—they would do 100 at a time! Lie face up on the ground with your arms over your head. In one fluid motion, bring your arms and legs up at the same time until your hands touch your feet. Come back down to the starting position.

Beginners: 5 to 10 seated V-ups.

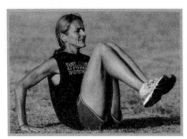 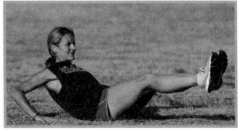

Intermediate: 15 to 25 seated V-ups.
Advanced: 30 to 50 pike-ups.

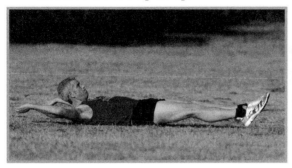 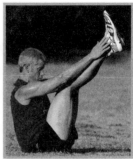

4. Cardiovascular: Mountain Climbers

These exercises will get your heart rate up in a hurry. Pretend you are less than one hundred feet from the top of Mount Everest. This is your last push to the top! Start in a push-up position, lying with your face down, your hands on the ground (or leaning on a table or desk), and your shoulders directly over your hands. Thrust your right leg up toward your chest while the other leg stays extended (almost in a jumping motion). Now alternate, extending the right leg and thrusting the left leg forward.

Continue as fast and furiously as you can for the specified time interval.

Beginners: Start with your hands on a table or desk for a greater angle; do 10 to 20 reps.

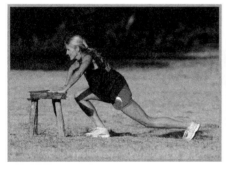 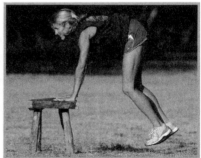

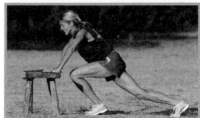

Intermediate: Start on the ground in the normal push-up position; do 25 to 35 reps.

Advanced: Start on the ground in a normal push-up position; do 40 to 50 reps.

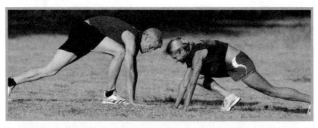

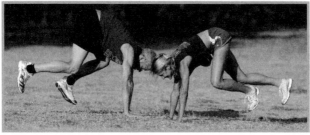

Warm Down

Let's go back and do 10 more meditative sun salutations from the Carl Sandburg stretching routine.

THERE! THAT'S THE E2 EXERCISE PLAN. Not so bad, is it? And if you get so good at these exercises you can do the advanced level for the full circuit, visit www.engine2diet.com fitness for more fun and exhilarating workouts that will challenge you still further.

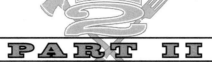

PART II

Making It
Work

1

THE **E2** ATTITUDE

In order to be accepted as a probationary firefighter by your new crew, you must show that you're willing to do whatever it takes. Your duties will be many and often tedious: You're expected to get to the fire station forty-five minutes before shift change and check the unit's supplies and medical gear; answer the phone after no more than two rings; wash the urinals and crappers; clean any dirty dishes and glasses lying around the station; lock up the station at night; be the first one out of bed after the 7:00 a.m. tone goes off; get the newspaper and place it on the kitchen table; make coffee for those who need stimulants to start their day; clean and wash the engine after morning cleanup; assist in all station tours; and order any needed supplies.

At the end of six months, if you're fortunate enough to pass your territory, policy and procedures, and firefighter exams, you will be welcomed into the firefighter fold with open arms and warm hearts as you begin one of the world's greatest jobs. Making it through these first six months can be a challenge, and having a positive attitude can make all the difference.

Similarly, your attitude will be your most important asset as you start the Engine 2 Diet. You, too, will have to be thick-skinned, because even some of your best friends may try to beat you down and get you to return to your old ways. You need to feel so good about the diet that you don't care what others say. After all, nobody on this planet cares about your own health as much as you should. Only you can take responsibility for your health. So if you want to be the healthiest person you can be, the E2 Diet is the way you should eat and don't let anyone tell you otherwise.

Over the course of the next four weeks, you will build character and determination as you become empowered by eating health-promoting and nutrient-rich foods. You will quickly realize how many of your friends, family members, and fellow Americans unconsciously throw piles of grease, suet, lard, and toxic waste into their precious bodies with a "This won't harm me" or "Why not live a little?" attitude that eventually bites them in the ass. Or heart. Or brain.

I firmly believe your attitude is the most important tool you have in life. With the right attitude, you can achieve anything—and I mean anything. So as you embark on the four-week E2 Diet, you will need to dig deep into your emotional closet, find your best attitude, and wear it for the duration of the program. Before long, you won't have to work at it. It will become a natural extension of your being.

Your first day on the E2 Diet will be the first day of the rest of your healthy, uplifting life. So get on board the Engine 2 fire engine and fire up for a great ride!

Here are some tips to keep your attitude positive and your motivation solid.

Find an E2 partner or friend. Nothing helps more than sharing the experience with someone else. Quite a few couples participated in the E2 Pilot Study, and it brought them closer as they made healthy meals—and avoided temptation—together.

Some years ago my wife, Jill, and I took a hike on the Austin Greenbelt, an eight-mile dirt trail that meanders next to beautiful Barton Creek. We invited co-firefighter and friend Matt Thomson; his wife, Erin; and Matt's parents, Reggie and Brenda.

We started the hike from the western trailhead, which begins with a steep one-half-mile-long downhill trek (nicknamed "the Hill of Life") to get to the part of the trail that runs along the creek. Matt and I ran and swam for close to an hour while Jill, Erin, and Matt's parents hiked around before we met them at the base of the Hill of Life for the hike back to our cars. Reggie and Brenda were whipped while Jill, who was carrying our four-week-old baby in a sling around her chest, was fresh as a daisy.

Reggie and Brenda decided right then and there to make some serious lifestyle changes. Matt and Erin enthusiastically recommended the Engine

MOTIVATION, BABY!

In 1994, I competed in my first Hawaii Ironman Triathlon, and I was all fired up—so much so that I came out of the 2.4-mile swim tied for first with three others, then took the lead biking up Palani Hill, which comes about a quarter of a mile after the swim. I was still leading for about 40 miles on the Queen Ka'ahumanu Highway when the forty-year-old triathlete legend, plant-powered Dave Scott, passed me, looking awesome. I had been racing for close to three hours, and amid all the excitement and action, what with the NBC cameras, helicopters, and motorcycles, I was having a difficult time controlling my pace and heart rate.

By the 56-mile turnaround in the little town of Havi, I was still in the top ten overall. Then, at about mile 70, it felt as if a pack of monkeys had jumped on my back. By mile 100 I was in big trouble. I finished the bike leg of the race by falling from 1st place to 224th. The thought of now having to run a marathon in the 100-plus-degree heat was nauseating, and I set out on what now felt like a death march. I ran and walked and suffered like a sick dog. Just remaining vertical was a chore. My feet swelled up in my shoes (the radiant heat off the black asphalt had reached 125 degrees) and I lost seven toenails. When I finally crossed the finish line, I looked up to see that I was the 567th overall finisher. And yet I did cross that finish line.

The lesson I learned: Always finish. I've competed in more than three hundred triathlons over the course of my career, and I've never failed to finish one. I remember Scott Tinley, one of the sport's legends, saying that he never quit in the middle of a race, because then it would be that much easier to quit the next time when things weren't going his way.

It's the same with this diet. Try not to surrender to your bad habits and temptations. Over the four-week period, the more you remain true to these guidelines, the less likely you are to fall back into your old ways later. Besides, you will soon see dramatic benefits, lose your cravings, and set up a successful pattern for life.

2 Diet, which they had just finished, so Reggie and Brenda decided to give it a whirl. Also joining up was their daughter Ashley, who was twenty-two years old at the time. Brenda was overweight and had been a Type 2 diabetic for a dozen years; Reggie and Ashley were overweight as well.

When Brenda completed the diet, her fasting blood sugar had decreased from over 200 to under 100, her A1C had dropped from 11.5 to 7.5, and she was able to stop taking all of her medications except one, a dose she now cut in half. She also lost 20 pounds, while Reggie and Ashley both lost 30—as a family, they lost a combined total of 80 pounds!

The Thomson family E2 partnership was a huge success because of teamwork and the unwavering support they showed one another. They are now eager to conquer the Hill of Life with their newfound weight loss and good health.

Your friend can be anyone in your life. For example, when Craig Walker was captain at station 3, he used to work with firefighter Arty Vasquez, who, when he wasn't at the station, managed Segovia Produce, one of Austin's best produce companies. Each week Craig compiled a list of all the fruits and vegetables he wanted, and Arty brought them to the station for him—some of the best produce in town at the best prices. Now that's a real E2 friend!

If you can't find a friend, find a book. Several E2 Pilot Study participants told me that though they had no social support, they found help in books. Obviously, there's no book I'd recommend more than the one you're currently reading, but for more support, check out my dad's book, *Prevent and Reverse Heart Disease*, Joel Fuhrman's *Eat to Live*, *Dr. Neal Barnard's Program for Reversing Diabetes*, or T. Colin Campbell's *The China Study*. Also, almost any book by Dr. John McDougall is of great help.

If you don't like books, go online. My site, www.engine2diet.com, is up, running, and ready to help you on your path to healthy eating.

Search out a support group in your community. Almost every community has its share of vegetarians, vegans, and health-conscious eaters; start aligning yourself with the like-minded. Find them through the internet, classifieds, or just by hanging around the local health food store.

Reframe your picture. I've been eating healthy for so long it's second nature. But for someone who's just starting out, it can be daunting to

Cindy Frost, 31

Firefighter

I knew when I signed up for the Engine 2 plan that the men at the fire station would give me a lot of crap. Many of them have big bellies and they're kind of proud of them—if they weren't, they'd have to do something about it. So they razzed me. But when no one else was around, many of them would come over and ask, "Did you really drop your total cholesterol forty points in two weeks? Would that happen to me?"

see your entire future consisting of food you don't know well. Instead, take it one meal at a time. Then, before you know it, that one meal will turn into two, two into four, four into eight, and boom! Soon you've finished the four-week program and realize, "Wow, that wasn't so hard. I love how I feel and I love the results!"

Be prepared to forgive yourself. We're all tempted by dietary devils now and then. So let's say that one day you can't resist temptation and you munch on a piece of devil's food cake. Don't beat yourself up over it.

During the E2 Pilot Study, one of the participants, firefighter Aaron Brooks from Station 23, went out one night with friends and ended up eating a big ol' cheeseburger. The next day she e-mailed me to say how sorry she was, how much she felt she had let me down, and that if I wanted to pull the plug on her participation, she would understand.

I wrote back and told her she had no reason to feel so bad.

So you crave a cheeseburger. If worse comes to worst, you eat it, then understand why you ate it, and then think about how it made you feel (bad!). The farther along you are into the four weeks, the more likely it is that, after eating that burger, you won't feel very good.

Two other E2 Pilot Study participants, Donna and John, occasionally fell into temptation. They were very successful on the diet (and both saw their LDL drop below 80), but every once in a while they knew they'd have to cheat, so they called it their "entertainment." If they decided to eat a cupcake, that was an entertainment. Instead of feeling guilty, they felt momentarily entertained.

Play to your strength. Some of you may already be really good cooks. If so, learn to be a great plant-based chef, like Craig Walker, the

THE ENGINE 2 RAZZ

We plant eaters at Engine 2 were ridiculed, berated, and teased mercilessly by firefighters from other stations. They said things like, "You guys don't eat food, you eat what food eats," or "You all have it easy, you don't have to cook. All you have to do is go out back and get some twigs and berries," or "Vegetarian is just an old Indian name for poor hunter."

In fact, after the media first spread the news about the plant-eating firefighters at Engine 2, we were inundated with mail from people all across the country; fans sent us cookbooks, chefs sent us food, several local vegetarian restaurants dropped off complimentary meals.

However, since few people understand the way the shifts work at a fire station, many of our new admirers visited us when the B shift, entirely composed of meat eaters, was present. Those firefighters grew tired of people telling them how wonderful they were for doing something they weren't doing.

To get revenge on us, B shift called the Texas Beef Council, which happily sent them an avalanche of brochures, posters, caps, T-shirts, and postcards, which the guys hung all over the station—and some of this meat-eating memorabilia is still around.

former captain at Station 3. When Craig went on the E2 Diet, I told him to use his culinary skills to his advantage—and boy did he, whipping up all kinds of dishes such as grilled Portobello mushroom and roasted red pepper sandwiches, black beans with Creole stir-fried cabbage, and fresh corn stir-fry with grilled BBQ tempeh.

Take strength from knowing how healthy you are becoming. Remember, in this country, one out of every three people is obese, and one out of every two will die of heart disease. You are now eating in such a way that you need never fear becoming a statistic—and will be free of the grip of the Western diseases that are debilitating so many Americans.

Take a test. Not everyone in every city has easy and affordable access to blood testing. But if it's available in your town, it can be a real help. Imagine how good you will feel when you see that after only two weeks of being on the E2 Diet, your cholesterol has dropped 20, 30, maybe even 40 percent. Your lethal LDL is falling. And your blood pressure is dropping. Your weight will be dropping, too. What better way to tell off the naysayers than by showing them hard-and-fast numbers? (You can read more about benchmarks and measurements in E2 Vital Signs, page 97.)

Keep healthy options handy. You don't want to find yourself craving a snack only to discover there's nothing in the cupboard. Carry something to nibble with you at all times, and keep healthy food handy in your office or car. One of the participants in the Engine 2 Pilot Study, Paul Koeningsman, carried a small cooler containing baby carrots, bell pepper slices, fruit, healthy crackers, and Fig Newtons everywhere he went. It paid off: His cholesterol went from 199 to 143, and his LDL from 98 to 35, and he tells me his painful diverticulitis came to an end.

AFTER LANCE ARMSTRONG raced his fifth and most difficult Tour de France in 2003, I received an email from him asking if I would help him with his diet.

I wrote back saying I would be happy to help. I also asked, "You want to win number six, don't you?"

"Do I want number six?" he replied. "Why do you think I'm asking you about this? Hell yeah, I want number six. More than I wanted number five actually. This year was not acceptable."

Not only do I love Lance's kick-ass attitude, but I also love that less than two weeks after his fifth victory, he was already thinking about the next one.

Is there something you'd like to improve in your life? Your performance? Your health? Your energy? Your longevity? Your weight? Make these goals a reality. Think about the sweet taste of success, and how good you will look and feel, inside and outside, in four weeks!

2

E2
VITAL SIGNS

How many people know their height and weight? Probably almost everyone. But how many know their total cholesterol, LDL cholesterol, HDL cholesterol, triglycerides, fasting glucose, blood pressure, and BMI? Probably very few.

I want this situation to change. You should be able to rattle off these numbers as easily as you do your address and phone number. These signposts are important clues as to the current state of your health and potential for disease.

Though we'll be talking about each of these markers individually, understand that all of them affect the others. If you see improvement in one area, more than likely you'll see it in others as well.

WEIGHT

One of the best parts of the E2 Diet is that you will lose weight in a sustainable, healthy, and permanent way. You will not be depriving yourself of any nutrients. Far from it—you will consume more nutrients than you ever have in the past. And you won't be hungry, because you can eat as many plant-happy foods as you wish.

However, this wonderful weight loss may not happen immediately—sometimes it can take up to two weeks for your body to transition to burning these cleaner fuels. Unlike some of the trendier diets that eliminate carbohydrates so you'll lose 10 to 15 pounds of water weight in the first two weeks, on E2 you'll lose real weight—i.e., fat, not just water—honestly and naturally.

So while you may lose only a few pounds or so a week for the first two weeks, the next two weeks should give you something to cheer about.

Check your weight regularly while on the plan; besides the joy you will feel as you watch the pounds drop, there is another advantage: If you are not losing as much as you'd like, it'll give you a chance to make a course correction. Pay careful attention to see if you are consuming too many calorie-dense foods, such as olives, avocados, peanut butter, nuts, smoothies, and fruit juices. These items can impede weight loss, and should be minimized or eliminated, depending on your goals.

For example, when thirty-six-year-old E2 Pilot Study participant McClain Sampson complained that she wasn't losing weight, I asked her to send me a one-week food log (see box), and I quickly saw that she was eating peanut butter, olives, and guacamole at almost every meal; i.e., she was simply substituting plant-based fats for animal ones. When we took these items off her menu, McClain lost 8 pounds over the next two weeks.

If you're trying to lose weight, but not succeeding as rapidly as you'd like, I recommend at least three cardiovascular exercise sessions, along with two E2 Functional Training sessions, a week (see The E2 Exercise Program, page 69). This will increase your resting metabolic rate (as noted, the rate at which you burn calories at rest). By exercising regularly, you can replace lazy fat with energetic muscle, burning calories at your desk or in bed as well as at the gym.

Some people actually lose too much weight on the E2 Diet—particularly men. At six feet, six inches, Jeff Brinker weighed 225 pounds when he started the diet. Over the next six months, he dropped down to below 185 pounds. So one night he called me, saying that he didn't want to lose any more weight (although he was thrilled that his cholesterol had dropped from 185 mg/dl to 111 mg/dl). I told him to consume more of the calorie-dense, plant-based foods McClain had been eating, and to drink smoothies and fruit juices and eat more whole grains and cereals. Soon enough, his weight was back to normal.

*   *   *

THE E2 FOOD LOG

A food log is a daily journal in which you write down every single thing you eat and drink during the day—breakfast, lunch, dinner, dessert, and especially snacks, as snacks are what often kill a diet.

My father first introduced me to the concept in 1985; he insisted that every one of his patients keep one, and every two weeks he would go over it with them to make sure they were correctly implementing the diet. These people kept this routine going for five years, so when you think twenty-eight days is a long time to keep a food log, think again.

Here's the way I like to do it: In a notebook, write in six columns that you fill in daily with your breakfast, lunch, dinner, snacks, daily activities, and observations. Find a time at the end of the day to write everything down, or better yet, make notes throughout the day so you don't forget anything.

For your convenience, feel free to sign up and keep one online at www.engine2diet.com.

Keep the food log for the entire twenty-eight days and it will give you some very valuable feedback—Am I eating enough leafy greens? Am I overdosing on breads and grains? Am I getting into a rut with my food choices? Am I skipping meals? Do the packaged foods I'm eating meet the E2 labeling standards?

I can't emphasize enough the importance of keeping a log for the whole twenty-eight days. Everyone in the Pilot Study—and I mean *everyone*—remarked on what an eye-opening process it was and how much junk they were unconsciously throwing into their systems.

For example, one participant remarked how the food log kept him honest; he knew if he drank a Coke or ate a piece of chicken he'd have to write it down, and that was the one thing that kept him from caving in. Another E2 participant ate oatmeal for breakfast, peanut butter and jelly for lunch, pasta for dinner, and a scoop of sorbet for dessert the entire first week. I told her I wanted her to diversify her foods; eat more fruits and more vegetables from every color of the rainbow. She agreed, started eating a larger variety of foods, and immediately enjoyed the different flavors and textures she hadn't even realized existed.

BEFORE YOU BEGIN THE FOUR-WEEK E2 DIET, please consider having the following tests done so you can track the dramatic changes that will occur as your body becomes healthier. And of course, talk to your physician about them.

TOTAL CHOLESTEROL

The average American has a total cholesterol above 200 mg/dl. The average American will also die of cardiovascular disease.

I'd like to see you aim to get yours below 150, even though your doctor may tell you that below 200 mg/dl is good enough.

It can be done, and done quickly. At the start of the E2 Pilot Study, the participants' average cholesterol level was 182. By the end, it was a heart-healthy 143.

LDL AND HDL CHOLESTEROL

As discussed, there are two types of cholesterol: LDL (low-density lipoprotein) and HDL (high-density lipoprotein). Your LDL is your *Lethal* cholesterol and your HDL is your *Healthy* cholesterol.

The average American has an LDL cholesterol level well above 100 mg/dl. But I don't want your LDL cholesterol to be average. I want your LDL to be E2 exceptional! As noted earlier, the magic number we're shoot-

McClain Sampson, 34
Graduate Student

The reason I did this wasn't for health. It was for my weight. I wanted to look good. If I look good on the outside, then I'll feel good on the inside. Maybe that sounds shallow, but I think a lot of women can relate. What I've discovered is that eating poorly is like casual sex. It feels really good and fun while you're doing it, but almost immediately afterward you have regrets and you have to start making contingency plans.

ing for on the E2 diet is below 80. Get your LDL below 80 mg/dl and you are essentially heart attack proof.

Some medical professionals stress the importance of the cholesterol risk ratio, which is your LDL cholesterol divided by your HDL cholesterol; the lower the ratio, the better—3.5 is generally seen as the cutoff between high risk and low risk.

I—and many medical experts—don't agree. Too many people take comfort in having a high HDL cholesterol level while their total and LDL cholesterol levels are in dangerous territory. The real goal here is to achieve a total cholesterol under 150 and an LDL under 80.

TRIGLYCERIDES

Even though I grew up in a medical household and was a triathlete for more than a dozen years, I had never heard of a triglyceride until the mid-1990s, when I started studying health and nutrition.

Triglycerides are fat globules in your bloodstream that many researchers believe are a high-risk factor for heart disease.

Just as your body needs a certain amount of cholesterol for cell repair, your body requires a certain level of triglycerides for fuel, particularly when it requires energy between meals or when you're exercising. However, too many triglycerides in your blood can be dangerous, as high levels have been shown to increase plaque formation, which as we know contributes to stroke and heart disease.

The goal, then, is to keep your triglyceride level under 150 mg/dl—the same as your ideal total cholesterol number.

Here are several ways to bring down elevated triglyceride levels:

a. Lose excess weight.
b. Eat whole, plant-based, high-fiber foods.
c. Exercise for thirty minutes a day.
d. Stop consuming excess calories—they're converted into triglycerides.
e. Watch your consumption of simple sugars such as alcohol, soda, honey, molasses, white flour, white pasta, and white rice.

FASTING GLUCOSE/BLOOD SUGAR

One of the best markers for checking whether diabetes is on your horizon is a fasting glucose test. Taken after you have fasted for twelve hours, this test will tell you the amount of sugar in your blood. A high fasting glucose number is an indication that your body is having a difficult time processing sugar.

A normal test result should be between 60 mg/dl and 100 mg/dl. If your level is over 125 mg/dl, you should consult your doctor.

On the E2 Diet, you can lower your fasting glucose level and even alleviate diabetes. For example, two E2 Pilot Study participants were Type 2 diabetics—one for five years and the other for twelve. Since going on the E2 Diet, both have been able to get off insulin, reduce their fasting blood sugars from over 200 mg/dl to under 100 mg/dl, eliminate or reduce all their oral medications, reduce their A1C levels from over 11 to under 7.5, and of course, watch their weight drop.

BLOOD PRESSURE

Your cardiovascular system consists of an amazing pump (your heart) and a set of pipes (your vessels). Every hour your heart pumps almost 70 gallons of blood to your 60,000 miles' worth of vessels.

Your blood pressure is a good indication of the health of your cardiovascular system. Unfortunately, almost one in three Americans has high blood pressure.

Blood pressure is reported as two numbers in the form of a fraction, such as 110/68. The upper number is called the systolic blood pressure and represents the force your heart exerts on your arteries when your heart squeezes. Systolic pressure should be 120 or below.

The lower number is called diastolic blood pressure, and represents the force the blood exerts on your arteries when your heart relaxes. That number should be 80 or below.

In America, we consider high blood pressure, or hypertension, to be a natural part of the aging process, but this doesn't have to be the case. In

---

E2 POP QUIZ

Q: Which of these foods has the highest percentage of saturated fat: butter, ice cream, steak, or cheese?

A: Cheese has the most saturated fat, at almost 20 grams of saturated fat per pound.

---

populations consuming a mostly plant-based diet, adults routinely have blood pressure levels similar to those of their children.

Thus, there is no reason why your blood pressure needs to increase as you age—unless you are consuming an animal-product-based diet, in which case it likely will go up, and you will have to go on medication to regulate it.

There are three main culprits of hypertension—the reasons eating animal-based foods is unhealthy.

The first bad guy is dietary cholesterol—if you eat animal-based foods, you're consuming a lot of cholesterol, which forms plaque inside your arteries, which in turn causes them to become narrow, forcing your blood pressure to rise.

The second is saturated fat, which attaches to the red blood cells, making your blood overly thick and sludgy, which in turn causes your heart to work harder. That, too, makes your blood pressure rise.

The third is excess sodium, which causes your body to retain fluids, which remain in your bloodstream. Once again, this condition asks your system to work harder, increasing your blood pressure.

How can you repair this situation? Eat the E2 way. There is no dietary cholesterol in plant-based foods. There is no saturated fat in plant-based foods (except coconuts). There is little sodium in plant-based foods. What could be easier?

BODY MASS INDEX (BMI)

BMI is the relationship between your weight and your height. With more than 64 percent of America overweight and greater than 30 percent considered obese, knowing your BMI may be the wake-up call you need to put down the pizza and remote control and pick up the banana and the walking shoes.

Too many Americans have become complacent with their weight and fall into a BMI category that places them at high risk for chronic disease. Recent studies have shown that the lower your BMI, the greater your chances of avoiding chronic Western diseases. Take care of yourself and get yourself down to a BMI that speaks to the seriousness of the obesity epidemic in America.

Visit www.engine2diet.com and use our handy BMI calculator, or find your BMI on the chart below and then take a moment to reflect on the dietary decisions you've made over the last ten years.

Keep in mind, though, that athletes and people with high muscularity (such as body builders) may have a BMI that indicates they are overweight when in reality their weight is healthy.

Weight in pounds

Height	120	130	140	150	160	170	180	190	200	210	220	230	240	250
4'6"	29	31	34	36	39	41	43	46	48	51	53	56	58	60
4'8"	27	29	31	34	36	38	40	43	45	47	49	52	54	56
4'10"	25	27	29	31	34	36	38	40	42	44	46	48	50	52
5'0"	23	25	27	29	31	33	35	37	39	41	43	45	47	49
5'2"	22	24	26	27	29	31	33	35	37	38	40	42	44	46
5'4"	21	22	24	26	28	29	31	33	34	36	38	40	41	43
5'6"	19	21	23	24	26	27	29	31	32	34	36	37	39	40
5'8"	18	20	21	23	24	26	27	29	30	32	34	35	37	38
5'10"	17	19	20	22	23	24	26	27	29	30	32	33	35	36
6'0"	16	18	19	20	22	23	24	26	27	28	30	31	33	34
6'2"	15	17	18	19	21	22	23	24	26	27	28	30	31	32
6'4"	15	16	17	18	20	21	22	23	24	26	27	28	29	30
6'6"	14	15	16	17	19	20	21	22	23	24	25	27	28	29
6'8"	13	14	15	17	18	19	20	21	22	23	24	25	26	28

Height in feet and inches

☐ Underweight ■ Healthy Weight ☐ Overweight ■ Obese

PERCENTAGE BODY FAT

Knowing your BMI is a good wake-up call, but knowing your percentage body fat can be a complete jolt. Carrying around excessive abdominal as well as visceral fat (which surrounds your internal organs) is a health hazard. It puts you at an increased risk for all kinds of diseases, from stroke and diabetes to cancer and heart disease.

The average male should have a body fat percentage of less than 20 percent, while a female's should be less than 25 percent. So when you realize that your body is 30, 40, or even 50 percent fat, it may finally light a fire under your ever-widening rear end.

Remember, muscle burns many more calories at rest than does fat. So the more fat and the less muscle you have, the fewer calories you need to maintain your weight, and the harder it will be to lose that weight.

Lose the dietary fat, start building muscle, and watch your body-fat percentage and pounds drop.

Many different methods are available for determining body fat, including using calipers and underwater scales. Whichever method you or your doctor use, for consistency you should employ the same one before and after you undertake the E2 Diet.

Our Pilot Study participants reported that one of their favorite parts of the E2 Diet was looking at their before and after body-fat numbers, and marveling that in just four weeks they had changed so dramatically.

THE 3-MINUTE HEART RATE STEP TEST

While fighting a fire, we can really get our heart rate going by doing something as simple as moving a charged house-line through a doorway, or breaking down a door with an ax. But often we'll need to recover very quickly, because at any minute we may have to carry out another heart-thumping task.

How quickly your heart rate drops, allowing you to relax and recover before your next effort, is a solid measure of its condition, as well as an indicator of potential heart disease.

A simple and yet effective test to gauge what kind of shape your heart is in is the 3-minute step test. First, take your resting heart rate. Find your pulse, either on your wrist or on your neck: Count the beats for 15 seconds, then multiply that number by 4. This is your resting heart rate per minute.

Next, find a stair or a box about 14 inches high. Step up onto the stair or box with your right foot, then your left, and back down, then start again with the right and then the left foot.

Continue stepping at an aggressive pace for 3 minutes, striving to get your heartbeat to within 80 percent of your maximum heart rate. A good formula for determining this number is to subtract your age from 220 and multiply the result by 0.8.

After completing the stair test, sit down and take your pulse again for 15 seconds, and multiply the number by 4. Now, wait 2 minutes and take your pulse yet again for 15 seconds. The larger the gap between the two numbers, the better.

For example, say your heart rate is 155 after doing the 3-minute stair test. After resting for 2 minutes, your heart rate is 120. The gap between the two is 35. However, if after 2 minutes your resting heart rate is 80, the gap is 75. Larger gaps mean your heart is better able to recover from strain.

Heart Rates			
Age	50 Percent	80 percent	Maximum HR
20	100	160	200
25	98	156	195
30	95	152	190
35	93	148	185
40	90	144	180
45	88	140	175
50	85	136	170
55	83	132	165
60	80	128	160
65	78	124	155
70	75	120	150
75	73	116	145
80	70	112	140
85	68	108	135

Maximum heart rates calculated at 220 minus your age

3

LABEL READING

The devil truly lies in the details. When you're eating a fresh peach, sucking on a messy mango, or polishing off an ear of summer sweet corn, you know exactly what you've got: a whole food product filled with the best and brightest Mother Nature has to offer.

The same cannot be said for anything that comes in a can, a box, or a package. These items can hold any number of dangers, from strange additives to heaps of fats—things that can destroy everything you've been working so hard to achieve. The only way to know exactly what you're eating is to learn to read the labels on these potential enemies.

So as you shop in the aisles of the grocery store, I want you to imagine yourself on your hands and knees, making your way through a pitch-black building where danger lurks behind every can, box, or package.

Luckily, you will be equipped with knowledge, the equivalent of a flashlight that will allow you to duck and weave your way through the potential hazards all the way to the checkout counter without a single scratch.

That knowledge will come to you in the form of labels. Labels are the ultimate test of whether a food is a true or false friend.

Let's begin with the two basic label-reading rules. I first heard them from a remarkable man named Jeff Novick, a former Kraft Foods major account manager who spent years convincing the public that they were buying healthy food products that, in reality, were unhealthy. Jeff now makes it his mission to teach people the truth about food companies, as well as how to read labels properly.

RULE 1

Never believe the claims on the outside of a package or box.

This includes such descriptions as "2 percent fat," "Reduced fat," "97 percent fat-free," "Fat-free," "Low in carbohydrates," "Healthy," "Wheat," "Natural," and many more assertions.

The food manufacturer's goal in using these terms is to lure you into purchasing their products. They could give a rat's rump about your health. All they care about is their bottom line—not your bottom, or any other part of you except your wallet. So they say whatever they need to say within the bounds of the law.

RULE 2

Read the nutritional information box as well as the ingredients list of every product.

Checking the facts is the only way to know what you are really putting into your mouth.

LET'S RETURN TO RULE 1 with some tips to make it easy to follow.

First, let's look at several examples of typical claims made on the outside of a package, box, or container; and learn how to decipher them.

2 Percent (or 1 Percent) Fat

A product's fat content is most accurately reflected using calories to determine the amount of fat. However, many companies use weight instead of calories. This spin factor can make a product appear to be 1 or 2 percent fat when in actuality it is 30, 40, 50 percent, or even more.

Comparisons based upon calories are much more relevant because our diet is based upon calories rather than weight—what nutritionist or scientist ever said, "You must eat at least eight pounds of food every day"?

Be very leery of products that claim to be 1 or 2 percent fat. Double-check by reading the nutritional label and determine the percentage of calories derived from fat.

For example, let's figure out the amount of fat in an eight-ounce glass of "2 percent" milk. The number of calories per serving is 120. The number of fat calories per serving is 45. If you do the math, this comes out to 37.5 percent fat. A far cry from the 2 percent most people think they are drinking! In case you're curious, 1 percent milk is about 25 percent fat, and regular whole milk is about 51 percent fat. That's the udder truth!

Here's the rule of thumb: To find the percentage of calories from fat in a product, first find the number of calories per serving. Then locate the calories from fat per serving.

Next find the grams of fat. To make the math easy, multiply 10 by the number of fat grams (a measurement of weight). This gives you the number of calories in each serving from fat. Lastly, divide fat calories by total calories to get the percentage fat per serving.

2 Percent Milk?

Nutrition Facts

Serving Size 1 cup 244g (244g)

Amount Per Serving

Calories 120	Calories from Fat 45
	% Daily Value*
Total Fat 5g	7%
Saturated Fat 3g	15%
Trans Fat	
Cholesterol 20mg	7%
Sodium 100mg	4%
Total Carbohydrate 12g	4%
Dietary Fiber 0g	0%
Sugars 12g	
Protein 8g	

Vitamin A	9%	•	Vitamin C	1%
Calcium	29%	•	Iron	0%

*Percent Daily Values are based on a 2,000 calorie diet. Your daily values my be higher or lower depending on your calorie needs.

SOURCE: Nutritional information from www.NutritionData.com

Fat Free or Nonfat

Did you know there are products in your house that are all fat, and nothing but fat, but are allowed to be labeled as nonfat? Namely, nonstick sprays such as Pam.

The manufacturer can label it this way because of serving size. The Food and Drug Administration allows any food with less than one-half a gram of fat per serving to call itself "fat free." This food industry trick is used to create all kinds of misleading labels.

In the case of nonstick spray, the manufacturers shrink the serving size down until there is less than one-half of one gram of fat per serving of the product (creating 702 servings per container). A serving that small is the equivalent of holding down the sprayer for one-third of one second! That's right—one-third of one second, which is physically impossible unless you have the lightning-fast reflexes of Bruce Lee.

Nutrition Facts
Serving Size 1 spray, about 1/3 second
1NLEA serving 0g (0g)

Amount Per Serving

Calories 2   Calories from Fat 2

% Daily Value*

Total Fat 0g	0%
Saturated Fat 0g	0%
Trans Fat	
Cholesterol 0mg	0%
Sodium 0mg	0%
Total Carbohydrate 0g	0%
Dietary Fiber 0g	0%
Sugars 0g	
Protein 0g	

Vitamin A	0% •	Vitamin C	0%
Calcium	0% •	Iron	0%

*Percent Daily Values are based on a 2,000 calorie diet Your daily values my be higher or lower depending on your calorie needs.

SOURCE: Nutritional information from www.NutritionData.com

Pam Spray—Fat Free or 100 Percent Fat?

Zero Trans Fat

Several food companies attempt to pull the wool over our eyes by making this wonderful-sounding claim in big, bold letters on the front of their packages. However, if you delve deeper by reading the ingredients list, about halfway down you'll often find hydrogenated oils hiding. (These produce trans fats, which I'll talk more about on page 116.)

For example, Mission Tortillas makes a good-looking wrap that advertises itself as having 0 trans fat (per serving). Turn the package over, and you'll see partially hydrogenated soybean oil (a source of trans fat) staring up at you, blushing. The claim takes advantage of that same FDA rule that allows food with fat to fib about itself.

Multigrain, Cracked Wheat, Seven-Grain, Stone-Ground, 100 Percent Wheat, Enriched Flour, Unbleached, Semolina, or Even Whole Grain Blend

Some of these claims can be genuine, but far too often they're not. Here's how to tell: A cracker, bread, or pasta is not really whole grain unless the first ingredient listed is "whole" followed by the type of grain. For example, whole oats, whole rye, whole wheat, whole semolina, or whole durum wheat.

The following are *not* whole grain products: semolina, durum, durum wheat, enriched durum wheat, bleached flour, unbleached flour, wheat flour, enriched wheat flour, and unbleached enriched wheat flour.

For example, Wild Oats makes a so-called "wheat cracker." The first ingredient is enriched wheat flour. That means this is not a whole grain cracker at all, but a processed, refined one. On the other hand, Ryvita makes a Rye and Oat Bran cracker. The first ingredient is whole grain rye flour. Excellent!

So keep your eye out for the word "whole" to ensure that what you're getting is truly a whole grain product.

Natural or Healthy

Too often, when you see the word "natural," it means someone is trying a little too hard to get your attention. Just because something is labeled as natural doesn't mean it's healthy.

For instance, Earth Balance makes a product they call a "natural buttery spread." They also claim it is "non-GMO," contains "expeller pressed oils," is "nonhydrogenated," and "100 percent vegan/non dairy." I'll have you know that 1 tablespoon contains 120 calories.

James Rae, 38

Firefighter

I was always a big ol' redneck. Ate a lot of steak, foods like that. I was basically a train wreck. My cholesterol level was 344 and I had a family history of heart issues—every male in my family except my dad died before the age of fifty-two, and my dad, at fifty-four, had a quadruple bypass. And still I ate whatever I felt like.

Then Rip and Josh and I decided to see who could lower their cholesterol the most, and we did it by eating nothing but plant-based foods. Mine went down to 196. That convinced me this was the way to go. But it's not just that my cholesterol level is lower, it's also that I *feel* cleaner. I truly believe that if someone like me can do it, anyone can.

And guess what? All 120 calories come from fat. You can put lipstick on a pig, but it's still a pig. You can dress up a buttery spread to look healthy, but if it's 100 percent fat, it's all fat.

As you can see, I was able to uncover the hype about numerous foods by following Rule 1: Never, ever believe the claims on the outside of a package or box.

If you're like me—someone who seldom has the patience to read instructions—I want you to take a deep breath and relax. Label checking can be a lot of fun, and within two to three trips to the grocery store, you'll find it will be a breeze.

WHEN READING THE "NUTRITIONAL FACTS" LABEL on a product, focus on four items, as stated in Rule 2:

The Number of Servings per Container

Does this product contain one, two, three, four, or seven hundred servings? You must first know this number to be able to estimate how many total calories, fat calories, grams of sodium, grams of fiber, and so on you are eating.

For example, a can of Amy's Organic Black Bean Chili has two servings per can, which is realistic given its size. On the other hand, a king-size Snickers bar has three servings per bar. Who eats one-third of a Snickers bar? With 170 calories per serving, that totals 510 calories per bar.

The same holds for a 20-ounce bottle of soda that claims to have only 100 calories per serving, but contains 2.5 servings per container, and thus actually has 250 calories. Remember our "fat-free" container of Pam, with 702 servings per container? Same principle.

Fat Content

When it comes to fat, food companies go even farther out of their way to make nutritional labels misleading. They use three different units (calories, grams, and percentages) on their labels, but never tell you exactly what percentage of the calories in that product come from fat.

The only way for you to know the percentage of calories from fat per serving is to divide the listed number of calories from fat by the total number of calories per serving. Instead, most people look at the percentage of total fat highlighted in the "Percent of Daily Value" section of the nutritional label, thinking that this number represents the food's total percent calories from fat content. It doesn't.

For example, that Amy's Organic Black Bean Chili can mentioned earlier has a total fat content of 2.0 grams per serving. Sounds almost fat-free, right? But 1 gram of fat contains a little more than 9 calories, or to make the math easy, we'll round that up to 10. Multiply 2.0 grams by 10 calories and you'll get 20 calories. This result means 20 calories of fat are in each serving.

To get the percentage of fat per serving, take the number of calories from fat per serving, divide it by the number of calories per serving, and multiply by 100. Amy's Chili has 20 calories from fat and 200 calories per serving, (20/200= .01x 100= 10%). The chili gets 10 percent of its calories from fat.

Remember, the E2 rule is to keep the total calories from fat in each food below 25 percent, and to find that, we divide the calories from fat by the total number of calories per serving.

Added No-No's: Sodium, Sugar, Fats

Companies list their products' ingredients in descending order by weight. The first ingredient weighs the most, the last ingredient weighs the least. Our goal is to avoid products that contain too much junk in the first half of the list.

Added Sodium

According to the National Academy of Medicine and the American Heart Association, the recommended sodium intake for adults is no more than 1,500 milligrams per day.

This may sound like a lot, but the average American actually consumes 4,000 milligrams per day. After all, just a teaspoon of table salt contains 2,200 milligrams.

Too much sodium in the diet is associated with hypertension (high blood pressure), a major risk factor for heart disease and stroke.

Take a look at the amount of sodium in some of the packaged, canned, and boxed goods in your home and you'll be blown away. For example, any can of commercially produced soup will have from 500 to 1,000 milligrams—per serving! And most cans contain two to three servings.

Here's an easy rule of thumb to control sodium: Limit the milligrams of sodium per serving to the number of calories per serving—and of course the fewer, the better.

Let's go back to our can of Amy's Organic Black Bean Chili with its 200 calories per serving. Check the nutritional label for sodium—you'll see that the can has 680 milligrams per serving. This figure is more than three times higher than we want (200 milligrams to match the 200 calories). And if you were to consume the whole can, which has two servings, you would be taking in 1,360 milligrams of sodium.

Added Sugars

Americans are overconsuming refined and simple sugars at an astonishing rate. This trend only contributes to the obesity epidemic and all the other diseases associated with it.

Sugars occur naturally in many foods such as fruits, vegetables, grains, and legumes. There's nothing wrong with these foods, despite their sugar content, as they are filled with fiber, vitamins, minerals, and nutrients.

However, when sugars are refined, adulterated, and processed, they become empty calories: They contain almost no nutritional value, can raise cholesterol levels, and make a beeline for your waistline.

These simple sugars can appear on a label as evaporated cane juice, evaporated cane juice syrup, sugar, brown sugar, fructose, high-fructose corn syrup, corn syrup, molasses, honey, barley malt, and beet sugar. Four grams of any of these devils is the equivalent of 1 teaspoon, which equals 16 calories.

Many people, especially kids, drink three to five sodas a day. Each soda has the equivalent of 10 teaspoons of sugar in it, meaning you're consuming 30 teaspoons of sugar (or 510 to 850 empty calories) if you drink three sodas a day.

Excessive sugar is found not just in snack foods, but in foods we rely on for meals. For example, it's difficult to find a boxed cereal that doesn't have four to six different types of sweeteners in the first half of the ingredient list. Kellogg's Low Fat Granola with Raisins lists five different types of sugar in the first half of its ingredient list: sugar, corn syrup, molasses, high fructose corn syrup, and malt flavoring. Cheerios, on the other hand, is a whole grain product and has just one sweetener: sugar. This is a better choice.

Still, my preference is that you eat a cereal containing no added sugars, such as Grape-Nuts or Bob's Red Mill Extra Thick Whole Rolled Oats, and add a natural sweetener such as sliced fruit. Now that's a winner!

Besides the number of different sugars found in food products, also bear in mind the quantity of sugars. As mentioned, 4 grams of sugar equals 1 teaspoon. Knowing this fact gives you a way to measure the number of teaspoons per serving. So when you look at the label of our Kellogg's Low Fat Granola with Raisins and see 18 grams of sugar per serving, just perform a simple calculation: 18 grams divided by 4, or 4.5 teaspoons of sugar per serving. Would you really sprinkle that much sugar on a bowl of plain flakes? I doubt it.

Added Fats

The first added fats to look for on a label are saturated animal fats. Saturated fats may include butter, eggs, lard, cheese, chicken fat, and/or beef fat. All are dangerous because they're major players in raising blood cholesterol levels and laying down plaque deposits.

Next, pay attention to added trans fats (trans fats are formed as a by-product of the hydrogenation process). You won't find the term "trans fats" listed in the ingredient list but they are produced in the manufacture of hydrogenated oils, so look for and avoid "hydrogenated" and "partially hydrogenated" vegetable oils in the ingredient list.

Trans fats are man-made gunk. Food companies take real vegetable oils, which are liquid at room temperature, and saturate them with hydrogen molecules to make them solid at room temperature—thus the term "hydrogenated."

The companies add these hydrogenated and resulting trans fats to bread, crackers, cookies, and other packaged goods to increase the product's shelf life (and decrease yours).

Trans fats, which should be avoided like the plague, have been implicated in raising LDL cholesterol and lowering HDL cholesterol, are a major contributor to plaque formations and heart disease, and promote cancers and tumors.

Last, sniff out hidden added fats such as monoglycerides and diglycerides. These substances go by fancy scientific terms, but they're fats and contain 9 calories per gram.

Food companies slide these into the ingredient list hoping you'll have no idea what they are. Steer clear.

Because fats are so prevalent, I'll give you some wiggle room by allowing you to eat products containing some fats, especially if they're minimal (appearing near the end of the ingredient list).

But I still draw the line that the total calories from fat in the product must represent no more than 25 percent of a food's total calories. Also make sure that any fats present are the healthier unsaturated ones rather than saturated or trans fats.

Back to our can of Amy's Organic Black Bean Chili: One of the ingredients is organic high oleic safflower and/or sunflower oil. I'm not a big fan of added oils. However, because this ingredient comes near the end of the ingredient list, and the total fat per serving of the soup is 10 percent, we'll approve this product, fat-wise.

When shopping, remember: The best sources of fat are whole foods, such as nuts, seeds, greens, grains, and vegetables, rather than added oils, meat, dairy, or man-made trans fats.

Heart-Healthy Olive Oil?

Nutrition Facts	
Serving Size 1 tbsp 14g (13g)	

Amount Per Serving	
Calories 119	Calories from Fat 119
	% Daily Value*
Total Fat 14g	21%
Saturated Fat 2g	9%
Trans Fat	
Cholesterol 0mg	0%
Sodium 0mg	0%
Total Carbohydrate 0g	0%
Dietary Fiber 0g	0%
Sugars 0g	
Protein 0g	
Vitamin A 0% • Vitamin C	0%
Calcium 0% • Iron	0%

*Percent Daily Values are based on a 2,000 calorie diet. Your daily values my be higher or lower depending on your calorie needs.

SOURCE: Nutritional information from www.NutritionData.com

Fiber

Fiber is a type of carbohydrate that your body can't digest, and therefore must expel. But that's good news!

Fiber rocks! It helps fill us up so we eat less. It keeps our gastrointestinal tract regular and our stools airy and light. It helps us to stabilize our blood sugar, maintain constant energy levels, and prevent disease.

Fiber acts like a little internal janitor, wielding scrub brushes that clean and then carry off disease-promoting substances such as cholesterol, throwing the nasty stuff in its garbage bag and hauling it to the dump.

Fiber is found exclusively in plant-based foods. One reason why the Engine 2 Diet recommends that you eat whole fruits and vegetables instead of drinking fruit and vegetable juices is because they contain fiber.

An eight-ounce glass of orange juice, for example, contains zero fiber, 120 calories, and 23 grams of sugar (giving you a huge glucose spike immediately followed by a bigger insulin rush). And it does little to satiate your appetite. Two oranges, on the other hand, give you 7 grams of fiber and 124 calories, don't cause the sugar and insulin spikes, and make you feel full. Ya!

Consuming a vast variety of fruits, vegetables, and legumes, as well as whole grain breads, cereals, and pastas, is the best way to reach your E2 Diet fiber goals. Most Americans consume between 10 and 15 grams of fiber per day. On the E2 Diet, we want you to get 40 to 50 grams.

THESE GUIDELINES ARE a lot to take in, I know. But now all that's keeping you from becoming a full-fledged, Cool Hand Luke, E2 label-reading pro is hands-on experience among the supermarket shelves. However, I have faith that the dangers lurking inside deceptive foods are now abundantly clear to you as you walk up and down the aisles looking for labels that pass the Engine 2 inspection test.

You no longer believe any of the claims on the outside of a package. You look for the number of servings per container and the amount of fat per serving. You are on the alert for added junk, such as sodium, sugar, and fats, and buy only high-fiber and 100 percent whole grain products.

You are a label-reading star.

BREAD

Here is a quick lesson on the difference between whole grain breads and the kind that have been pillaged.

The anatomy of the wonderful whole grain:

Bran: The outer layer containing most of the fiber as well as healthy amounts of protein and B vitamins.

Germ: The nutrient-rich embryo containing vitamins E and B and protein.

Endosperm: The fluffy inside, which is 83 percent starch. This is all that remains after the bran and germ are removed—and this is what white bread is made of.

What does this mean? It means 100 percent whole grain has 97 percent more vitamin E, 78 percent more fiber, 78 percent more magnesium, 82 percent more vitamin B6, 80 percent more selenium, 58 percent more copper, and 37 percent more folacin than white bread!

4

MAKING IT WORK FOR LIFE!

hen I developed the Engine 2 Diet, my mission statement was: Educate and motivate people to eat a plant-strong diet so they can enhance their lives and avoid the common killer diseases.

I am now inviting you to become part of this mission. Start just by putting one foot in front of the other. One meal at a time, one day at a time; string them together, several days in a row, and soon enough your first week will be over. Before long you'll have your sights set on the finish line.

Although the plan outlined in this book is a twenty-eight-day diet, it is my hope that this is just the beginning of your plant-strong journey. And as on any journey, you may stumble and fall. That's okay. It's even expected. No one gets it right the first time—or the second. I've been tweaking and adjusting this plan for more than three decades myself.

The goal is to keep working on it. Continue to expand your knowledge base, cooking skills, and recipes, and watch your confidence grow until there's no stopping you. Soon enough, the E2 lifestyle will be second nature, you'll be firing on all cylinders, and you'll wonder how you ever used to eat all that other stuff you once called food.

In fact, you will be living the dream—feeling great, looking terrific, and free of the common modern ailments that compromise and debilitate so many lives. This dream is easily within your reach.

While you're living it, I want you to learn to love the plants that are giving you back your life. I want you to see the brilliance of apples, oranges, blueberries, broccoli, black beans, yams, whole grains, kale, and all of nature's other wonders. When it comes to food, these are the winners, the unsung heroes that deserve all the credit, the foods that have your best interests at heart. Don't let anyone tell you otherwise.

I want to tell you one last thing. You are a champion. Just by reading this book, you're moving from second-class to first-class foods, from nutritional excess to nutritional excellence. You now know more about nutrition than 99 percent of the world. You are on your way to a plant-blessed life.

I am rooting for your success and want the very best for you. I also look forward to hearing about your progress at www.engine2diet.com. Write me! Maybe your story will be featured in my next book.

Now get out there and earn your health!

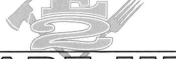

PART III

Recipes and
Meal Plans

INTRODUCTION

his part of the book will allow you to bring the E2 way of living and eating into your home. Get ready to spoil yourself silly with dynamic plant-based foods, and by the end of the twenty-eight days, the Engine 2 plant-strong way of life will be second nature to you.

You'll start with the most basic of tasks, which means going to the grocery store to buy all the wonderful healthy E2 foods that will soon be bursting out of every crack, cupboard, and pantry of your home.

Next, I want you to pay close attention to all the E2-recommended kitchen tools and cooking ware. Having the proper equipment will make your life in the kitchen as streamlined as possible. Over a weekend, take the time to transform the tools and the foods in your kitchen, and over the next twenty-eight days your body will reward you with a transformation of its own.

You'll also be reading time-saving tips; suggestions on easy, delicious, and nutritious snacks; and some simple yet effective storage ideas that will help you maximize the life of your new-bought foods.

Then, for those of you who love to cook, this next section should make you very happy: dozens of recipes for eating the E2 way. These wholesome, healthy foods will soon make you wonder how you ever got along without them!

For those of you who don't love to cook, have no fear. You can thrive the E2 way simply by eating out intelligently, snacking wisely, and buying prepared foods sensibly. Several of the E2 Pilot Study participants barely knew what a kitchen was, and they did just as well as the cooking-loving plant-eaters. For more information on how to do this, please check out the E2 website, www.engine2diet.com.

So get psyched for fun and adventure as you prepare, cook, and, best of all, eat a whole new array of exciting plant-tasty foods. Throw yourself with reckless abandon into the kitchen and watch as everything within your circle of influence—except your waistline—starts to expand: your health, your food, your confidence, your awareness, and your spirits.

TRAVELING AND EATING OUT

It's always easier to eat well on your home turf. That's why when you're not home, I want you to pay special attention to staying on top of your E2 Diet game plan.

PLAN AHEAD

Spend a few minutes packing a separate carry-on bag of foods that travel well: healthy sandwiches, oranges, apples, plums, grapefruits, carrots, bell peppers, cherry tomatoes, raisins, whole grain bagels, walnuts and almonds, and Engine 2 hummus. This will keep you away from airline snacks and convenience store junk.

PACK WHAT YOU CAN

Whenever I travel, tucked securely in my suitcase is a Tupperware container filled with my Rip's Big Bowl cereal (see page 150); some healthy store-bought dried soups that simply require hot water; fruits; vegetables; healthy baked chips; salt-free whole grain pretzels; and one or two of the healthier energy bars.

ADAPT AND OVERCOME

If you didn't have a chance to plan ahead, don't rationalize your way into eating poorly. Go for the healthiest option available. Search out healthy options such as fruits, nuts, seeds, vegetables, and whole grain crackers. Also consider fruit Newtons, whole grain bagels, subs, veggie pizza, veggie burgers, and salad bars.

EATING OUT WISELY

Be courageous and ask for what you want—even if it's not on the menu. I don't care if it's a five-star restaurant or a taco stand, make a smart substitution—beans and/or potatoes for meat, extra vegetables for cheese, tofu for chicken. Ask politely and the server will move mountains for you: "Make mine a burrito supreme but hold the steak, cheese, and sour cream, and double up on the beans, veggies, and potatoes. Thank you very much."

Some cuisine-specific tips:

Italian: Order bread and ask for roasted garlic or a side of marinara sauce for dipping.

Chinese, Japanese, Thai: Order vegetables with tempeh, tofu, or wheat gluten over brown rice or whole grain noodles.

Mexican: Order bean or veggie tacos, enchiladas, or burritos topped with a healthy salsa. Ask for warm corn tortillas to dip into salsa in place of fried chips.

American: Order a baked potato with no extras (such as sour cream, butter, or bacon bits), a big plate of steamed vegetables, and a side salad with balsamic vinegar or salsa for dressing.

Pizza: Ask for whole wheat crust with extra tomato sauce, no cheese, and tons of vegetables.

Everywhere: Avoid soda. Instead, request a large glass of water with a side of sliced lemons or limes to squeeze into it.

Dessert: Order a healthy sorbet or fresh fruit. Stay away from the pies, cakes, and ice creams!

GET CREATIVE

Pack a cooler for your car if you're on a road trip. One E2er recently told me about one you can plug into a car or regular electrical outlet to keep food cold. See if a local grocery store can deliver to your hotel room. Call room service and order several vegetable side dishes off the menu along with a plate of rice and make your own veggie stir-fry.

USE THE INTERNET

Surf for sites such as www.HappyCow.net, www.VegGuide.org, or www.VegDining.com, which will help you find all the vegetarian, vegan, and plant-based restaurants within a two- to ten-mile radius of wherever you are.

KEEP UP THE ATTITUDE!

If you're motivated, you'll plan ahead, pack what you can, adapt, ask for what you want, use the internet, be creative, and consistently overcome many of the temptations lurking everywhere you turn. You'll feel empowered, not defeated, when you return home feeling as wonderful and centered as when you left.

1

GETTING YOUR KITCHEN IN E2 SHAPE

just as you're getting yourself into great shape, you'll want to get your kitchen in shape, too. Let's start by stocking your pantry and cleaning out your kitchen.

Make sure that you always have a variety of fresh, whole foods on hand. This includes fruits, vegetables, whole grains, legumes, and healthy snacks. Here is a breakdown, from your pantry to your freezer.

E2-APPROVED FOODS
TO KEEP IN YOUR PANTRY

Cold Cereals (Found in Conventional Grocery Stores)

Arrowhead Mills
>   Puffed Corn
>   Puffed Kamut
>   Puffed Millet
>   Puffed Rice
>   Puffed Wheat
>   Shredded Wheat

Barbara's Bakery
> Multigrain Spoonfuls
> Shredded Wheat

Kashi
> 7 Whole Grain Nuggets
> 7 Whole Grain Puffs

Nabisco Shredded Wheat

Nature's Path
> Kamut Puffs
> Millet Puffs
> Rice Puffs

Post
> Grape Nuts
> Shredded Wheat
> Uncle Sam Original Wheat Berry Flakes

Hot Cereals (Found in Conventional Grocery Stores)

Arrowhead Mills
> Bulgur Wheat
> Oat Bran
> Oat Flakes
> Original Plain Instant Oatmeal
> Steel Cut Oats

Bob's Red Mill
> 5, 6, 7, 8, and 10 Grain
> Barley Grits
> Creamy Brown Rice
> Creamy Buckwheat
> Organic Kamut
> Rolled Oats
> Whole Wheat Farina

McCann's Irish Oatmeal

Quaker
Barley
Instant Oatmeal
Oat Bran
Old Fashioned Oats

Pasta and Grains

Ancient Harvest
Polenta
Quinoa
Quinoa pasta

Eden Quinoa

Kashi Pilaf

Lundberg Family Farms
Brown rice
Wild rice blends

San Gennaro Foods Polenta

Uncle Ben's Instant Brown Rice or Boil-in-Bag Whole Grain Rice (10-minute cook time)
Whole wheat pasta is available in most store brands.

Any brown rice, quinoa, or corn pasta is also acceptable (as long as only the single grain is listed in the ingredients). And, there's also an extraordinary amount of gluten-free pastas out there made from black beans, red lentils, chickpeas, and mung beans, to name just a few.

Whole Grain Breads/Tortillas/Pizza Crusts[1]

Alvarado Street Bakery
Oil-free breads and bagels
Sprouted Wheat Tortillas

---

1. *Since some of these do not meet the 1:1 sodium rule, you should make sure that if your bread is higher in sodium, your entire meal profile is low in sodium and you do not add salt to the overall meal.*

Bremner Food Group
Natural Ry-Krisp-Fat Free

Dave's Killer Bread
Powerseed
21 Whole Grains and Seeds
Blues Bread

Food for Life
Ezekiel 4:9 Bread
Ezekiel 4:9 Sprouted Whole Grain Tortillas

Garden of Eatin'
Bible Bread (regular and salt-free)

Great Harvest Bread Co.

Mestemacher
Muesli Bread
Natural Three Grain Bread
Organic Rye & Spelt Bread
Whole Rye Bread

Nature's Hilights
Brown Rice Pizza Crust

Pure Grain Bakery
Gourmet Rye Bread
Pumpernickel Bread

Ryvita Crispbread

Wasa Crispbread
Hearty
Lite Rye
Multi Grain
Sourdough

What to look for at Whole Foods
(Whole Foods Brand Foods)

*Breads/Tortillas**

Engine 2 Plant-Strong Crispbreads
Original
Seeds and Spice
Triple Seed

Engine 2 Plant-Strong Tortillas
Brown Rice Tortillas
Sprouted Ancient Grains Tortillas

Engine 2 Plant-Strong Stone Baked 100% Whole Wheat Pizza Crusts

Engine 2 Plant-Strong Sprouted Ancient Grains Burger Buns

Whole Foods 365
Organic Fat-Free Tortillas

Canned Beans

Whole Foods 365
No-salt-added canned beans
Organic no-salt-added beans
No-salt-added boxed beans

Cereals

Engine 2 Granola
Apple Pumpkin
Blueberry Vanilla
Plain Jane

Engine 2 Rip's Big Bowl
Banana Walnut
Original
Triple Berry Walnut

---

* Most corn tortillas are also E2-approved.

Engine 2 Rip's Power Up Bowl
Double Berry (hot cereal)
Original (hot cereal)

Whole Foods 365
Bite-Size Wheat Squares
Organic Corn Flakes
Organic Multigrain with Flax Instant Oatmeal
Organic Oats and Flax Instant Oatmeal
Organic Old-Fashioned Rolled Oats
Organic Original Instant Oatmeal
Organic Quick Oats
Organic Steel Cut Oats

Condiments

Engine 2 Hummus
Roasted Red Pepper
Traditional

Whole Foods 365
Ketchup
Low-Sodium Soy Sauce
Mustard

Plant-Based Milk

Pacific
Original Oat milk
Vanilla Oat milk

Whole Foods 365
Organic Unsweetened Almond Milk
Organic Unsweetened Soy Milk

Frozen Food

Engine 2 Grain Medleys
Ancient Grains Blend
Fiesta Blend

Morning Blend
Wild Rice Blend

Engine 2 Plant Burgers
Italian Fennel
Pinto Habanero
Poblano Black Bean
Tuscan Kale White Bean

Engine 2 Ravioli
Chickpea and Spinach
Butternut Squash and Kale
Mediterranean Vegetable
Cannelloni and Kale

Engine 2 Pizzas
Vegetable Pizza
BBQ Pizza
Green Supreme Pizza

Engine 2 Burritos
Ranchero
Spicy Green Chili
Vegetable

Whole Foods 365
Brown rice
Frozen fruit (all varieties)
Frozen vegetables (all varieties)
Green chickpeas
Quinoa

Pasta

Whole Foods 365
Brown Rice
Whole Wheat Pasta
Pasta Sauce

Engine 2 Pasta Sauce
Classic Tomato Basil
Red Bell Pepper Marinara

Salad Dressings/Dips

Health Starts Here Dressings
Balsamic
Balsamic Fig
Caesar
Garlic Tahini
Sesame Ginger

Salsa

Whole Foods 365
Salsa (look for lowest-sodium options)

Soups/Broths

Engine 2
Firehouse Chili
Moroccan Style Stew
Vegetable Stock

E2-*NOT*-APPROVED FOODS TO REMOVE FROM YOUR KITCHEN

I'm not saying you have to throw these foods out—but I've found that if bad foods are in sight, you're more likely to eat them. So I recommend that if you don't want to toss them, at least store the nonperishables in a closet, ask a neighbor to hold on to them, or donate them to a worthwhile organization. Keep in mind the old adage: Out of sight, out of mouth.

The foods you'll think about tossing are all the animal-based products, oils, and canned and packaged goods that contain more than 2.5 grams of fat per 100 calories.

All food (canned, boxed, frozen) containing more than 2.5 grams of fat per 100 calories.

Meat: All foods containing meat, animal fat, or meat stock.

Dairy: All foods containing dairy, including cheese, milk, yogurt, butter, ice cream, sour cream, and coffee creamers.

Cheese substitutes: They contain too much fat and sodium, and many include casein, a dairy protein.

Oil: All foods containing oil, including mayonnaise, salad dressing, olive and canola oils, and sauces.

Refined sugars and high-fructose corn syrups: Mixes, sauces, sodas, candy, and cookies.

Processed grains: White flour, white rice, and white pasta.

TOOLS TO KEEP IN YOUR KITCHEN

The items below can be found very affordably at your local next-to-new shop.

Knives: butcher, paring, and tomato
Serrated spoon
Spatulas—one for flipping pancakes and tofu, one for scraping
    mixing bowls
Wooden stirring spoons
Soup ladle
Salad tongs
Long-handled tongs (just the thing for tortillas and roasting peppers)
Potato masher
Garlic press
Citrus squeezer (handheld)
Grater/zester (microplane)
Measuring cups
Measuring spoons
Cutting boards
Colander
Sieve (perfect for smaller grains such as quinoa)

Steamer
Three mixing bowls: small, medium, large
Canisters (for storing rice, oats, cereals, and legumes)
Storage containers (Tupperware and Ziploc-type bags)
Pans with lids (large skillet, soup pot, saucepan)
Baking sheet
Casserole dish
Muffin tin
Loaf pan
Rice cooker
Blender
Cuisinart-type food processor
Mini-Cuisinart (optional, for small jobs and easy cleanup)
Immersion blender (for soups—inexpensive and well worth it)
Toaster oven (for bread, sweet potatoes, wraps, corn in the husk)

HANDY E2 KITCHEN TIPS

Cutting, Slicing, and Chopping

Leave the skins on your vegetables for maximum nutrition. Most skins are edible and delicious, but make sure to scrub them first to remove dirt, wax, and pesticides.

Chop and slice vegetables, onions, and root vegetables into different shapes for a more interesting presentation and varied taste. Beets, for example, can be sliced into thin or thick circles, diced into cubes, or shredded raw for salads and garnishes.

Smaller shapes cook more quickly. For example, take care not to cook shredded carrots for as long as you would carrot circles.

Stir-Frying

Stir-frying is the process of cooking food quickly in a superheated skillet or wok. Ingredients are added in rapid succession, with just a few stirs after each one. The finishing touch is either Bragg Liquid Aminos, low-sodium tamari, or a homemade mirin sauce. At E2 we are really crazy about our mirin sauce as superb enhancement to our stir-fries. To make it, use a few tablespoons of mirin (a Japanese sweet wine); a tablespoon of low-sodium tamari mixed with a tablespoon of citrus juice; a teaspoon of sweetener; and a few teaspoons of cornstarch.

Combine these sauce ingredients in a small bowl and add them to the cooking vegetables just a minute before you remove the vegetables from the heat. Cook and stir for a moment or two until the al dente (slightly firm) vegetables are coated with the thickened, savory sauce.

Sautéing

Engine 2 foods are not sautéed in the traditional way (in a pan swimming with olive oil or butter). At the firehouse we always started with a hot pan and a few drops of water. We liked to sauté with low-sodium vegetable broth, orange juice, carrot juice, or simply water. At home, Jill and I also like to use wine and beer (the station is alcohol-free).

Steaming

Steaming is a great way to enjoy your vegetables! Buy a little steamer basket. Place it in a soup pot or large skillet and fill with enough water to barely reach the bottom of the steamer basket. Once the water is boiling, toss your washed produce into the basket and cover the pot with a lid. Take care not to overcook. Super fresh vegetables, or those cut into small pieces, cook very quickly.

Caramelizing Onions

Onions contain sugars that are released when they are sautéed until slightly brown. We cook ours on high heat for 5 to 7 minutes. Stir the onions continuously in a skillet with a few drops of water until they begin to brown. A teaspoon or more of dark brown sugar, maple syrup, or molasses can be added at this stage to speed the process along and complement the onions' natural flavor. Stir for another 1 to 2 minutes. The sweet and savory flavor of caramelized onions is delicious as a base for soups and stews, as well as on salads and veggie burgers.

Grilling Vegetables

Vegetables, fruits, tofu, and other meat substitutes are delicious when cooked over coals or a wood fire. For the best grilling, choose plants that contain a lot of water so they won't dry out. When grilling carrots and potatoes, be sure to wrap them in foil to prevent them from shriveling up. Next, choose plants whose bold flavors will complement the smoky goodness of the open flames; bell peppers, corn on the cob, onions, squash, and pineapple are among my favorites.

Don't forget about the fungi and bread, either. Mushrooms sizzle like few other foods. A good Portobello mushroom brushed with BBQ sauce, a pinch of salt, and plenty of black pepper makes one heck of a great "burger." Also, a simple dough of whole wheat flour, salt, water, and yeast can be grilled to make an awesome flatbread. Finally, have some non-oil salad dressing or marinade on hand to keep your veggies moist if they start looking a little parched. Spray the bars of the grill with a nonstick spray, or employ one of those neat-o perforated skillets or cooking baskets atop the coals or flame.

Remember, one of the many great things about plants is that they contain zero HCAs (heterocyclic amines), carcinogens linked to higher rates of colorectal, pancreatic, breast, and prostate cancers, which are abundant in all meats when grilled. So, if you want to have your cake and eat it, too, grill your veggies—all char, no carcinogens!

Using Homemade Vegetable Stock

This is a great way to maximize your produce purchases. Rinse vegetables and greens thoroughly to avoid getting any sand or dirt in your stock. Place discarded trimmings (stalks, root tips, tomato hearts, vegetables that are past their prime but not rotten, the tough inside shell of onions, greens, ends of carrots, etc.) into a stockpot with water to cover. Add a few bay leaves, 1 teaspoon whole peppercorns, and 2 peeled cloves of garlic. Cook covered for 20 minutes. Save the stock liquid, and discard the boiled trimmings and seasonings. Stock will keep covered in the refrigerator for a week, and indefinitely in the freezer.

A Quick Tip on Beans

We often use canned beans to save time, but you can easily cook your own instead. Look through dried beans for any small pieces of dirt or rock. Then rinse them thoroughly in a few batches of water and soak overnight. The next morning drain and boil one part dried beans with three parts water (i.e., 1 cup of beans with 3 cups of water) in a large covered soup pot on low heat for two hours. Check on them a few times, stirring to make sure they're not sticking, and add water as necessary. Lentils cook quickly, in 45 minutes or less. Kidney beans take the longest time to become tender. Cooked legumes keep well in the freezer to be thawed for future use.

Warming Tortillas and Wraps

At the firehouse, we warmed our tortillas and wraps directly on the big gas burners, using a pair of tongs to turn them. Wraps can also be warmed in a dry skillet until they puff in the center.

For a warm wrap that is soft and pliable rather than toasted and puffy, place it in a cloth towel and microwave it for 30 seconds.

Toasting Nuts and Seeds

Nothing could be simpler than home-toasting nuts, plus you can be assured there is no fat added when you roast them yourself. Nuts and seeds change in flavor and texture when they are roasted in a dry skillet or oven, or toasted in a toaster oven. Stir them constantly, taking care not to let them burn. Add them to soups and salads, or use them as a garnish for stir-fries and vegetable dishes.

Roasting Peppers and Fresh Chilies

Toast peppers on a gas flame, over the grill, or in a hot skillet until the skins are blackened and puffing away from the peppers. Make sure the peppers are evenly toasted, then peel the skins away from the flesh under running water. Cut peppers in half and remove the seeds and veins. Slice into strips. Make extras and freeze for future use.

Preparing Mangoes

Hold the fruit in your hand so a flat side faces your palm. Slice the fruit in half laterally, running the knife next to the seed, then use the knife to score the flesh into cubes. Invert the scored mango and cut the cubes away from the skin with the knife.

Preparing Avocados

Slice the fruit in half lengthwise, running the knife around the seed. Pull the pieces apart. One section will still have the seed attached. Hit the seed with the sharp side of the knife so the knife is lodged in the seed, and then give the knife a quarter turn, and the seed will pop out. Then score and cube the meat, and use a spoon to scoop out the insides.

Preparing Leafy Greens

Remove those thick stems magically from collard greens and kale: Hold the stem firmly in your dominant hand. Loosely hold the lower part of the stem just below the leafy greens in the other hand. (With some kale, you may need to tear back the lower leaves to expose some of the stem.) Holding firmly with the dominant hand, curl your other hand into a fist and then slide it up the spine. You are left with all the greens in your opposite hand and the bare stem in your dominant hand. (Collard stems do not always come away as far up the leaf, but that doesn't matter.)

Now you should have a pile of greens that are easy to chop into bite-size pieces. Don't waste the stems: They are full of fiber! Assemble them in a row and chop into tiny pieces. Add them to soup or use them in homemade stock.

E2 POP QUIZ

Q: How much fiber is in a glass of milk, a slice of chicken, and an organic egg?

A: Zero. There is no fiber in any animal foods. Fiber is found only in plant foods.

E2 SUBSTITUTIONS

Meat substitutes: Tofu, made from soybeans, is a hearty and very malleable food. Think of it as a blank slate, an excellent substitute for fish, chicken, cheese, cream, eggs, and mayonnaise. Tofu packed in water should be drained before using.

Tofu can be either soft or hard. Soft, or silken, tofu blends into a smooth cream and is excellent in desserts. Hard, or firm, tofu retains its shape, and can be sliced or crumbled. All tofu is about 40 percent fat (except for low-fat versions).

Firm or extra-firm tofu can be drained and then pressed firmly with a cloth to remove excess water. Crumble, slice, or dice it, and add it to the skillet for a spin with your favorite vegetables and seasonings.

Marinate tofu the way you would chicken or fish—with herbs, citrus juice, cracked black pepper, vinegar, wine, or low-sodium tamari or soy sauce. Cook marinated tofu in a skillet, under the broiler, or on a grill until it is nicely browned on both sides.

Try freezing a drained block of tofu. After it thaws, frozen tofu soaks up marinades easily since it becomes more porous in the freezing process. It also changes slightly in consistency, becoming chewier.

Seitan is a wonderful substitute for chicken or beef, and comes in both flavors. Derived from wheat in a process that extracts the gluten or wheat protein, it slices and dices easily without falling apart, and is delicious plain.

Tempeh is a form of fermented, unprocessed tofu; it is remarkably nutritious. It usually comes in hard bricks that can be sliced or chopped, then added to stir-fries or chilies.

Salt: Instead of salt, season with lime juice, lemon juice, plenty of salt-free spices, low-sodium tamari, Bragg Liquid Aminos, vinegars, tomato juice, low-sodium soy sauce, or vegetarian Worcestershire sauce.

Sweeteners: Use pure maple syrup, molasses, unrefined dark brown sugar, fruit juice, mashed bananas, or applesauce.

Dairy and butter: Try sliced bananas and fruit and no-oil-added nut butters on toast in place of butter. Use blended lite soft silken tofu in recipes in place of sour cream and milk.

STORAGE TIPS

Greens

Lettuces and leafy greens will keep much longer if you take a few minutes to prepare them for the refrigerator. Fill the sink with cold water and separate the leaves from the head. Remove any brown bits. Allow the greens to soak for a few minutes or longer to rehydrate them. Layer them in dish towels or paper towels and place them in your refrigerator's vegetable crisper.

Evert-Fresh bags, available at grocery stores and online, are invaluable for keeping greens (as well as fruits and vegetables) fresh and crisp.

Avocados and Fruits

Guacamole, avocado slices, and peeled or sliced fruits will keep their beautiful color if you store them in airtight containers or plastic bags with a dash of lemon or lime juice. Keep the mother seed in with leftover avocado or guacamole to help prevent its turning an ugly shade of green.

Nuts, Nut Butter, and Flaxseed Meal

These items will last longer without becoming rancid if refrigerated.

Cook Fresh!

Make sure your spices, baking powder, and flours are fresh for optimal flavor and results.

TIME-SAVER TIPS

- Prechop vegetables and fruits, and store them in airtight containers in the fridge or freezer.
- Freeze cherry tomatoes as easy additions to any recipe.
- Make extra brown rice, quinoa, and other whole grains for wraps and leftovers. Store in the refrigerator up to a week.
- Make an E2 spread at the beginning of each week.
- Make an E2 salad dressing at the start of each week.
- Double tofu recipes, and keep cooked tofu for a quick snack or addition to wraps, salads, and tacos.
- Double muffin and pancake recipes, and freeze the leftovers—they are just as delicious when rewarmed a week later.
- Buy a one-gallon Tupperware or similar-type container and toss in a dry salad, which will last for days.
- Boil water immediately when you start preparing dinner so you don't have to wait 5 to 7 minutes before adding pasta, grains, vegetables, or potatoes.

2

E2 EASY WEEKLY PLANNER

The E2 Easy Weekly Planner is a flexible outline that allows you to pick and choose meals from the E2 Recipes section and plug them into the Weekly Planner as you see fit.

Most people prefer to start the diet on a Monday, so in general, Day One will be a Monday and Day Seven will be a Sunday. However, feel free to start whenever you'd like.

To make it work, all you have to do is check the Weekly Planner category for that day's meal, and then go to E2 Recipes and find it. For instance, for breakfast on Day One, for an E2 Hearty Cereal Bowl, you may choose to have Rip's Big Bowl (page 150). For lunch, it's an E2 sandwich; you might pick the E2 Basics Open-Faced Sandwich (page 164). Then, for your comfort plate, perhaps the Mac-N-Cash (page 207), with the Fruit Bowl with Soy Drizzle for dessert (page 249).

The Weekly Planner follows a simple pattern: The weekday breakfasts can be whipped up in less than 3 minutes, while the weekend breakfasts such as pancakes or omelets require some preparation and cooking time. The weekday lunches require zero cooking time, and take merely 3 to 5 minutes of preparation time—or if you decide to make your lunch from last night's dinner leftovers, just the time it takes to grab something out of the refrigerator and a fork. (I always encourage people to make more than they can eat at dinner so they have the option of leftovers for lunch or the following dinner.)

The dinners are broken up into nine different categories of familiar foods with a healthy twist, such as pizzas, pastas, soups, salads, burgers, Tex-Mex favorites, and stir-fries. There is always something for everyone. For example, on pasta night, if you don't like mushrooms, you can steer clear of the Mushroom Stroganoff (page 193) and dive into Bow Ties with Pesto (page 196). Or if on comfort food night you don't care for Mac-N-Cash (page 207), you can settle into Shepherd's Pie (page 206).

To get started, some people like to pick out seven dinners from the first week, make a corresponding list of groceries, head over to the grocery store, and get everything needed to last the week.

EASY WEEKLY PLANNER

The ENGINE 2 DIET

	BREAKFAST	LUNCH	DINNER	DESSERT
DAY 1	Hearty Cereal Bowl	Sandwich	Dinner Plate	Fruit Selection
DAY 2	Fruit & Toast	Lunch Salad	Pasta or Pizza	Chocolate Indulgence
DAY 3	Hearty Cereal Bowl	Wrap or Pita	Soup or Big Salad	Fruit Selection
DAY 4	Fruit & Toast	Lunch Salad	Tex-Mex	Cobbler, Cookies, or Pie
DAY 5	Hearty Cereal Bowl	Sandwich	Burger & Fries	Fruit Selection
DAY 6	Saturday Special	Wrap or Pita	Stir-Fry	Pudding or Mousse
DAY 7	Sunday Morning Pancakes	Sandwich, Pita, or Leftovers	Comfort Dinner	Cobbler, Cookies, or Pie

Leftovers from dinner make a great next-day E2 lunch either on a bed of mixed greens, in between pita bread, or over brown rice. Personally, I've gone several days in a row feasting on E2 dinner leftovers that are often better the next day after all the flavors have had that extra time to marinate.

3

E2 RECIPES

E2 Breakfasts / 149

    E2 Hearty Cereal Bowls / 150

    E2 Saturday Specials / 152

    E2 Sunday Morning Pancakes and Muffins / 157

    E2 Fruit and Toast / 162

E2 Easy Lunches / 163

    E2 Sandwiches / 163

    E2 Wraps and Pitas / 168

    E2 Lunch Salads / 172

E2 Dinners / 175

    E2 Dinner Plates / 177

    E2 Burgers / 184

    E2 Potato Sides / 190

    E2 Pasta / 192

    E2 Pizza / 196

    E2 Comfort Dinners / 201

    E2 Stir-Fries / 208

    E2 Big Salads / 212

    E2 Soups / 217

    E2 Tex-Mex Favorites / 222

E2 Dressings, Spreads, and Marinades / 232

E2 Desserts / 245

    E2 Chocolate Knockouts! / 245

    E2 Fresh Fruit and Fruit Bowls / 248

    E2 Cobblers, Cookies, and Pies / 250

    E2 Puddings and Mousses / 255

Growing up, I hated vegetables. The only ones I would eat were peas and corn. I'd make bacon, lettuce, and tomato sandwiches without the lettuce and tomato, and double up on the bacon and mayonnaise. But over the last thirty years, I've grown to appreciate and love vegetables, beans, and whole grains, along with the art of cooking them.

To relax your spirit and strengthen your health, following are more than 125 mouthwatering recipes filled with the foods I now love, and love to serve friends. In fact, every guest who has eaten a plant-hearty meal at our home or at Engine 2 has declared, "I never knew plant-based food would taste this good! I'd eat this way if I knew how."

Well, now you'll know how. Grab the ingredients, follow the instructions, and you're off to the races with a smile!

E2 BREAKFASTS

Breakfast is my second-favorite meal of the day, right next to dinner. It comes after a forced fast of six to eight hours (unless you've been sleeping at the firehouse, where more likely than not you've been up three times between midnight and dawn), when the body begins revving up its metabolic engine.

Too many people forgo breakfast because they're in a hurry, don't have an appetite, or are trying to lose weight. But if you skip breakfast, your body will enter conservation mode and slow down your metabolism in an attempt to conserve energy—a bad move if you're trying to lose weight.

So make breakfast a priority. Some of these recipes require just 2 minutes to prepare, roughly the same amount of time that elapses between the moment we hear the alarm at the station and when we arrive at the scene of the incident.

E2 Hearty Cereal Bowls

Most of the cereals on the grocery store shelves are loaded with processed junk and should be avoided—they're candy in a box. I want you to fill up your morning cereal bowl with whole grains containing little to no added sugar. Start your day with a bang rather than a misfire!

Rip's Big Bowl

This has been my mainstay breakfast for almost thirty years. I never get sick of it and no two bowls are ever quite the same, depending on which fruits are in season and the plant-based milk I have on hand.

This was also a favorite recipe for most of the E2 Pilot Study participants. As a seven-year-old daughter of one of the participants said, "I look forward to waking up in the morning just so I can have my Rip's Bowl."

Let your appetite be your guide as to the size of your bowl.

¼ cup old-fashioned oats
¼ cup Grape-Nuts or Ezekiel 4:9 nuggets
¼ cup bite-size shredded wheat
¼ cup Uncle Sam cereal
1 tablespoon ground flaxseed meal
2 tablespoons raisins
½ handful of walnuts
1 banana, sliced
1 kiwi, sliced
1 grapefruit
¾ cup plant-based milk

Toss all ingredients except the grapefruit with the plant-based milk in a bowl. Cut the grapefruit in half and use a small, sharp knife to remove the segments. Add the segments to the top of the bowl and squeeze in the juice. Top the bowl with plant-based milk.

Variations:

In a pinch, simply add water (the fruits blend with the water and give it a sweet taste).

Add any fresh or frozen fruit, such as peaches, cherries, mangoes, blueberries, or red grapes.

If you want to lower your cholesterol levels even more, use half a cup of oats and omit one of the quarter cups of the other cereals.

E2 Hot Lap Bowl

When Engine 2 pulls up to a house fire, our lieutenant immediately does a "hot lap"—a 360-degree walk around the structure to determine the scope of the situation before deciding on a course of action.

Experiment with different ingredients to personalize your bowl and determine the best plan of attack.

1 cup uncooked hot cereal (see E2-Approved Foods to Keep in Your Pantry, page 127)
1 tablespoon ground flaxseed meal
2 tablespoons raisins or dried cranberries
1 banana, sliced
½ cup fresh or frozen fruit
½ cup plant-based milk
½ handful of walnuts

Cook cereal in water according to package directions. Once the cereal is finished cooking add the ground flaxseed meal, raisins, banana, and fruit, and stir. Drizzle with the plant-based milk and top with walnuts.

Simple Cereal Bowl

There's something really nice about a plain bowl filled with one type of cereal, whether it's Grape Nuts, oat bran flakes, or plain oats, and a little fruit. So, bring breakfast down a notch and enjoy the simplicity.

1 cup whole grain cereal (see E2-Approved Foods to Keep in Your Pantry, page 127)
1 banana, sliced, or any other fresh or frozen fruit
½ cup soy milk

Place the cereal in a bowl, and top with fruit and soy milk.

Quick Oatmeal Bowl

A warm, healthy breakfast doesn't get any easier than this bowl, which I discovered through an old Canadian triathlete friend named Dan Murray. Dan was one of the best Olympic distance triathletes of the early 1990s; he was the first man to run a sub thirty-minute 10K in a triathlon. Now that's quick!

1 cup old-fashioned oats
1 cup water
1 banana, sliced
1 tablespoon molasses

Place the oatmeal, water, and banana into a large bowl and stir. Microwave on high for 2 minutes. Top with molasses and serve.

E2 SATURDAY SPECIALS

One morning at the fire station, I woke up at seven and saw Derick walk past wearing just his pants.

"Did you sleep with your pants on?" I asked.

"Yes," he said. "I always do when I'm driving."

"Is that so you're a little faster to the draw?"

"No," he said. "It's to remind me where I am."

I know exactly what he's talking about. Sometimes you wake up and you have no clue where you are or what's going on. So when that alarm goes off at 3:00 a.m., if you can look down and see that your pants are on, this might just give you the edge you need to do your job that much more efficiently. At other times, of course, just having a great breakfast is all you need to get going.

These breakfasts are intended to serve two, but they can easily accommodate one: Simply cut the amounts of every ingredient in half and enjoy.

French Toast

French toast takes me back to slow Saturday mornings sitting around the Esselstyn family table and the feel of powdered sugar on the roof of my mouth. Serve this deliciously healthy version of French toast with pure maple syrup and fresh fruit.

Serves 2

1 banana, mashed
½ cup plant-based milk
1 teaspoon vanilla extract
½ teaspoon cinnamon
4–6 slices whole grain bread or baguette

Combine the banana, plant-based milk, vanilla, and cinnamon in a shallow bowl. Dip the bread slices in the mixture and cook in a skillet on medium heat for 2 minutes on each side, or until lightly browned.

Variations:
Serve with a light sprinkling of powdered sugar for that roof-of-the-mouth taste.

Migas Especiales

I've never met a Texan who doesn't like migas. The word is derived from the Spanish word for crumbs, and the dish is traditionally made using eggs, cheese, sausage, tortillas, and salsa. Part of the Tex-Mex food culture, it's a dish that creates a very satisfying harmony of tastes. Served with a side of healthy refried beans, corn tortillas, salsa, and fresh fruit, with this dish mornings just don't get much better.

Serves 2

1 onion, chopped
8 ounces mushrooms, sliced
2 tomatoes, chopped
1 pound firm tofu, drained, pressed with a cloth, and mashed
1 teaspoon turmeric
7 corn tortillas: 3 cut into 1-inch squares and 4 to make little tacos (or en-
    joy the way you would toast)
Salsa (see page 240)
16-ounce can fat-free vegetarian refried beans, warmed in skillet or micro-
    wave
1 cup fresh fruit

Sauté the onion with a few drops of water in a skillet on medium heat for 5 minutes or until translucent. Add the mushrooms and tomatoes. Cook for 7 minutes or until most of their juices have been cooked away. Add the tofu, turmeric, and tortilla squares. Cook for a few minutes, or until the mixture is warmed through. Place a generous spoonful of migas on a plate and top with salsa. Serve with a side of beans, the remaining tortillas, and the fresh fruit.

Breakfast Tacos

I don't know if it's just a Texas thing, but breakfast tacos are very popular in the Lone Star State. They're fast, easy, and really good. We warm up corn tortillas on the gas burner, throw in the filling of the day, and top them off with salsa. No breakfast taco would be complete without salsa.

Serves 2

½ cup cooked black beans
8 ounces frozen fat-free hash brown potatoes
6 corn tortillas
Salsa (see page 240)

Sauté the black beans with a few drops of water in a skillet on medium heat for 5 minutes. Set aside. Add a little water to the pan, turn the heat up to high, and sauté the hash brown potatoes for 7 to 10 minutes, or until golden brown. Spoon ingredients into warm tortillas. Top with salsa.

Variations:
Try black beans with avocados, or scrambled tofu or hash browns with refried beans.

Make your own refried beans and hash browns by mashing and cooking extra beans and potatoes from dinner.

E2 Omelet

I know that many people find it hard to leave eggs behind—but each egg is 67 percent fat and has over 212 milligrams of cholesterol. This is not good if you're looking to lose weight and clean out your arteries. That's why I've included this healthy and tasty recipe. Topped with salsa, it's a real winner.

Serves 2

Omelet Filling
8 ounces mushrooms, sliced
½ onion, diced
1 red bell pepper, sliced into strips
1 cup baby spinach

Omelet
Nonstick spray
12 ounces firm tofu
2 tablespoons soy milk
2 tablespoons nutritional yeast
2 tablespoons Ener-G egg replacer
1 tablespoon vital wheat gluten
2 teaspoons Bragg Liquid Aminos
¼ teaspoon onion powder
¼ teaspoon turmeric

For Serving
Salsa (see page 240)
Fresh fruit

For Omelet Filling:
Sauté the mushrooms and onion in a large skillet with a little water over high heat for 5 to 7 minutes or until the mushroom liquid is mostly gone. Remove to a bowl and return the skillet to the heat. Toss the bell pepper strips in the skillet and cook for 3 minutes, until they begin to brown slightly. With 1 minute remaining toss in the baby spinach. Remove from heat and set aside.

For Omelet:
Blend together all the omelet ingredients until smooth. Spray a large skillet lightly with nonstick spray and pour half of the batter into the center, using a spoon to spread it out evenly over the bottom of the

skillet. Turn the heat to medium. Cover and cook for 8 minutes, then place half of the cooked filling in a line down the center of the omelet. Use a spatula to flip both sides over the veggies, cover, and cook an additional 2 minutes. Remove from heat and gently shake the skillet from side to side a couple of times to loosen the omelet. Carefully slide the omelet onto a plate. Repeat with the second half of the batter and the rest of the filling. Serve immediately with salsa and a side of fresh fruit.

Variations:
Add sliced avocado, diced tomatoes, pineapple chunks, or sliced olives.

E2 Sunday Morning Pancakes and Muffins

Sunday mornings offer a wonderful opportunity to gather with family and friends for a breakfast pancake bonanza. Warm up the griddle, get out the spatula, and start whipping up some good old-fashioned flapjacks. At the firehouse we took great pride in flipping pancakes as big as manhole covers—without even using a spatula. The trick is a quick flick of the wrist, perfect timing, and a deft catch with the cast iron skillet.

Lemon Cornmeal Pancakes

We generally make these on Sunday mornings when things are slow, which gives us time to cook up and eat these great pancakes. We found this recipe in a wonderful cookbook called *Vegan with a Vengeance* by Isa Chandra Moskowitz. We then ramped up the nutrition by using whole wheat flour instead of white flour and omitting the oil.

Serves 3 to 4

1 ¼ cups whole wheat flour
2 teaspoons baking powder
½ teaspoon salt
¾ cup cornmeal
2 cups plant-based milk
½ cup soy or almond yogurt
Zest and juice of 2 lemons

Mix the dry and wet ingredients in separate bowls. Add the dry ingredients to the wet ingredients, stirring to remove lumps. Cook according to the directions for E2 Basics Pancakes (see page 158).

E2 Basics Pancakes

At least once a week we took turns making pancakes at the station. We keep three or four varieties of Arrowhead Mills pancake mix in the freezer at all times: multigrain, oat bran, buckwheat, and cornmeal. We top our pancakes with applesauce, fresh fruit, a plant-based yogurt, maple syrup, or a thin layer of peanut butter (unless you're like Matt Moore, who doesn't like peanut butter but loves cashew butter).

Serves 2

1 ¼ cups pancake mix
1 ¾ cups water or plant-based milk
Nonstick spray

Combine the mix and the liquid in a large bowl, stirring to remove lumps. Heat a dry skillet until a drop of water dances on its surface. Spraying the skillet once with nonstick spray should allow for three batches of pancakes. Ladle a large scoop of batter into the pan. Several pancakes can be cooked at once if you're using a large skillet. Cook until the batter begins to bubble and the bottom of the pancake is golden. Flip and cook on the other side until both sides are golden.

Variations:

Add bananas, blueberries, peaches, or strawberries with walnuts or pecans to the batter. Or sprinkle 70 percent pure cocoa chips into the batter for a chocolate treat!

Spelt Blueberry Pancakes

This recipe was created by one of the Engine 2 participants, Anthony Salerno, who makes these for his daughter, Ella. He then freezes the leftovers for future quick breakfasts or late-night snacks. This recipe is for a double batch.

Makes 25 to 30 pancakes

2 cups spelt flour
2 cups oat flour
¼ cup ground flaxseed meal
2 tablespoons baking powder
½ teaspoon salt
3½ cups plant-based milk
¼ cup applesauce
2 tablespoons maple syrup
1 tablespoon vanilla extract
2 cups blueberries

Whisk the flours, flaxseed meal, baking powder, and salt together in a large bowl. Combine the plant-based milk, applesauce, maple syrup, and vanilla in another bowl. Form a well in the center of the dry ingredients and add the wet ingredients. Stir the batter just until the dry ingredients are thoroughly moistened; it will seem very thin, but it will thicken.

Let the batter rest for 15 minutes (spelt flour takes a little longer to absorb liquids). If you can't wait, your pancakes won't be as crisp. After the batter has rested, fold in the blueberries. Cook according to directions for E2 Basics Pancakes (see page 158).

Mighty Muffins

These are the brainchild of my friend Bridget's brother, Michael. An amazing cook and a Buddhist, Michael travels internationally as a chef for his teacher and others in the Buddhist community.

Once cooled, these muffins keep well in the refrigerator for a week. Eat them cold or warm them briefly in the oven.

Makes 6 large muffins or 1 enormous loaf

3 cups oat bran flakes
1 teaspoon baking powder
½ teaspoon salt
¼ cup maple syrup
1 large apple, grated
6 brown bananas, lightly mashed (leave some chunks)
Juice of 1 lemon
¼ cup walnuts, chopped or cut in half
¼ cup raisins
¾ cup water

Preheat the oven to 400°F. Line a large muffin tin with parchment paper. Combine the bran flakes, baking powder, and salt in a large bowl. In another large bowl, combine the maple syrup, apple, bananas, and lemon juice. Add the walnuts, raisins, and water. Combine the wet and dry ingredients in one bowl and stir for 1 minute. Pour the batter into the prepared muffin tin and bake for 22 to 25 minutes or until golden brown on top.

Variations:

Bake the batter in a loaf pan lined with parchment paper, and enjoy hearty slices instead of muffins.

Add three thinly sliced pears or 1 cup of 70 percent pure cocoa chips to the batter.

Quick Bran Muffins

Yes, these come out of a box, but that's okay. There's no harm in relying on great products made by quality food companies—especially when they are quick and delicious.

Makes 6 small muffins or 2 small loaves

7-ounce box bran muffin mix (we like Hodgson Mill)
2 ripe bananas, mashed
½ cup water

Preheat the oven to 400°F. Line a small muffin tin or two mini loaf pans with parchment paper. Mix the ingredients together and spoon the batter into the prepared tin or pans. Bake for 25 minutes or until a toothpick inserted in the center comes out clean.

Variations:

Add extras to the batter! Consider:

1 teaspoon Ener-G egg replacer mixed with 1 tablespoon water
1 diced apple or pear
6 ounces blueberries or raspberries
½ teaspoon vanilla extract
½ cup raisins

Rip's Tip

Make a double batch of these muffins and freeze half of them for a quick, on-the-go breakfast or a healthy snack.

E2 Fruit and Toast

I'm going to harp on this until I'm blue in the face: I always want you to use 100 percent whole grain toast, bagels, or English muffins. I particularly like the Ezekiel 4:9 brand whole wheat bread, which you can keep in the freezer. Simply throw a couple slices into the toaster while you're getting out the jam or nut butter or slicing up some fruit to place on top. Pull the toast out of the toaster, add your toppings, and head out the door.

PB and Banana

Serves 2

4 slices whole grain bread
1 tablespoon no-oil-added peanut butter
2 bananas, sliced

Toast the bread. Spread slices thinly with peanut butter. Top with sliced bananas.

Variations:

Substitute bagels or English muffins for bread. Use any no-oil-added nut butter in place of peanut butter. Add E2-approved jam or preserves. Use any sliced fresh fruit in place of bananas.

Fresh Fruit Extravaganza with Mint

Go to town! Use cantaloupe, honeydew, grapes, grapefruit, kiwi, strawberries, oranges, mangoes, watermelon, or blueberries.

Serves 2 to 4

Every fruit in your kitchen, sliced, diced, or chopped
Zest of 1 lime
Juice of ½ lime
Juice of 1 grapefruit
Sections of 1 orange
1 bunch mint leaves, chopped

Toss the fruit in a bowl with zest, juices, and mint.

For a surprisingly zingy pleasure, try a squeeze of lemon on your fruit—especially on slices of watermelon.

E2 EASY LUNCHES

One day Austin firefighter Brad Mendenhall from Station 8 traveled to Station 2. "Just because," he said, "I'm dying to eat some of your healthy vegetarian cuisine."

The battalion chief, who overheard him, said, "Well, then, all you have to do is go out into the front yard, pick up some twigs and leaves, throw them in the skillet with some oil, and you're set."

The battalion chief was not an E2er.

I replied that we wouldn't be using any oil. The chief then called me a freak.

I told Brad to ignore the peanut gallery and introduced him to several Engine 2 favorite lunches that are especially easy to prepare.

E2 Sandwiches

Each shift in the Austin Fire Department lasted twenty-four hours. At Engine 2, we were called the C shift, which means that at noon the crew was always either coming to work to relieve the B shifters, or getting off and waiting for the A shifters to relieve us.

As hectic as lunchtime could be, what with all shifts joining in, the meal had to tide us over until dinner, when we could sit down to a solid, three-course plant-based feast.

Derick Zwerneman, 35
Firefighter

My first day at Station 2, I got up early and made blueberry muffins. They smelled great, but when everyone else came down to the kitchen, they said, "Huh, lot of calories in those."

I thought, "Who are you jerks?" No one had told me about how healthy Engine 2 ate.

At the time my menu planning was simple—I used to see what meat was for sale and then my wife and I would plan our meals around that. If pork chops were on sale, then it was pork chops for dinner. Now that we eat a plant-based diet, we're more creative. And our palates have changed, too. I used to love chicken. Today the smell of it makes me kind of sick.

E2 Basics Open-Faced Sandwich

Years ago, when we were short on time, we'd run to a nearby sub shop and order the number 11 without the cheese and mayo, and ask them to double up on all the vegetables. Eventually, we'd just say, "An Engine 2." But then a new owner took over and rescinded the half-price discount for firefighters and police officers. So we started making the Engine 2 at Engine 2.

Serves 2

4 slices whole grain bread, toasted
E2 spread of choice
1 cucumber with skin on, scrubbed and sliced into thin rounds
1 large tomato, sliced
1 handful arugula
1 cup alfalfa sprouts
Lemon pepper to taste (we like the Mrs. Dash brand)
Lemon or lime juice

Spread one side of each piece of bread thickly with the E2 spread. Top with vegetables, arugula, and sprouts. Season with lemon pepper and a squeeze of lemon or lime juice.

Variations:

Top the sandwich with chopped cilantro, green onions, salad greens, avocado, shredded raw beets, or shredded carrots.

Ann's Panini with Hummus, Mushrooms, and Spinach

At the firehouse we have great old cast iron skillets that weigh as much as concrete bricks. They come in handy because the key to making a fantastic panini is to get a hefty amount of weight on top of the sandwich as it cooks. You can prepare this in one of two ways: Place an iron skillet (or other heavy object) on top to smush the sandwich, or be decadent and purchase a panini maker and use as directed. I got one for Christmas. It sears perfect lines on top of the bread. You'll know it's ready when the hummus drips over the sides like melted cheese, the outside is crispy, and the inside is soft.

This dynamite recipe comes from my mother, Ann. And by the way, for those of you who don't know, a panini is an Italian sandwich.

Serves 2 (or one ravenous firefighter)

8 ounces mushrooms, sliced
Low-sodium tamari or Bragg Liquid Aminos to taste
4 slices whole grain bread
Healthy Homemade Hummus (see page 236)
4 green onions, chopped
½ cup chopped cilantro
2 handfuls baby spinach

Sauté the mushrooms on medium heat in a skillet for about 5 minutes or until soft. Season lightly with tamari. Spread all four bread slices thickly with hummus. Sprinkle two pieces of the bread with green onions and cilantro and reserve the other two pieces as sandwich tops. Using a slotted spoon to allow any liquid to drain away from the mushrooms, place them on top of the green onions. Put a handful of spinach on top of the mushrooms. Top the two sandwiches with the reserved pieces of bread, and press to seal.

Carefully place the sandwiches in a skillet on medium heat. Place a heavy casserole dish on top of the sandwiches to flatten them. Cook the weighted sandwiches on one side for about 5 minutes, taking care not to let them burn. Flip the sandwiches and cook the other side in the same way. When done, paninis will be quite thin and browned on both sides.

Plant-Strong Brats

These bratwursts are the brainchild of Renee DeMan, a super enthusiastic and spirited Whole Foods Market store team leader at the Spring Lake Wall store on the New Jersey shore. Renee, who attended an Engine 2 seven-day immersion program in 2012, told me it took her two years to perfect this creation. I was skeptical. A plant-strong brat that doesn't have oil, plant protein isolates, or a ton of salt—and it's really good? All I have to say is these are insane! Insane! The brown rice spring roll wrappers meld into the filling and create a brat that any German would be proud to serve.

Makes about 7 brats

Base Ingredients
>   15-ounce can garbanzo beans, rinsed and drained
>   15-ounce can pinto beans or black beans, rinsed and drained
>   1 cup rolled oats
>   ½ cup cooked brown rice (see E2 Brown Rice, page 175) or riced cauli-
>   flower

American-Style
>   3 tablespoons diced fresh tomato
>   3 tablespoons diced green or red bell pepper,
>   3 tablespoons diced red onion
>   2 tablespoons mustard
>   2 tablespoons diced pickles or low-sodium pickle relish

Mexican-Style (use black beans instead of pinto beans)
>   2 tablespoons Salsa (see page 240)
>   2 tablespoons diced green chilies
>   2 tablespoons chopped cilantro
>   2 tablespoons diced green or red bell pepper
>   1 cup shredded zucchini or squash

For Wrapping
>   7 brown rice spring roll wrappers

Process the base ingredients in a food processor for 30 seconds, until ingredients are mixed well and the consistency of the inside of a sausage. (If you are looking for a good arm workout, you can mash the ingredients using a large spoon.) Transfer the mixture to a large bowl and add all the filler ingredients for either the American- or Mexican-Style brats, stirring to combine. Place the bowl in the refrigerator for 15 minutes.

When the filling mixture has chilled, fill a shallow bowl with warm water. Working one at a time, dip a spring roll wrapper into the water to soften it, and then lay it flat on a clean work surface. Place ⅓ cup of the filling in the center of the wrap in the shape of a hot dog and then fold up the wrap and bring in the sides. Chill the rolled brats for another 10 to 15 minutes.

To cook on the stovetop, place the brats in a skillet on medium-high heat and cook for 5 to 7 minutes, rotating every 1 to 2 minutes. To cook on the grill, rotate every 1 to 2 minutes until the wrapper starts to bubble.

Kale, Lemon, and Cilantro Sandwich

Sometimes I don't know what I'd do without the creative genius of my amazing, enthusiastic, brilliant mother! Ann serves this one open faced on toasted bread. You won't believe how good a superhealthy sandwich like this can taste until you try it! Gene Stone, my co-writer and one of the Engine 2 participants, hated kale before tasting this sandwich. Now he's a devoted kale, lemon, and cilantro sandwich eater.

Any greens will work. The lemon adds an almost sweet taste. Be generous with it!

Serves 2

1 bunch kale, rinsed and drained
Zest and juice of 1 lemon
4 slices whole grain bread
Healthy Homemade Hummus (see page 236)
4 green onions, sliced
½ bunch cilantro or parsley, chopped
1 lemon with skin on, sliced into very thin rounds

Tear the kale leaves away from the thick stems (see Preparing Leafy Greens on page 140). Discard the stems and chop the leaves into bite-size pieces. Fill a pot with about 4 inches of water and add the kale. Bring to a boil, cover, and cook on low heat for 2 to 3 minutes, until the kale is tender. Check frequently.

When the kale is tender, drain well. Shake the strainer so all the water is gone, then sprinkle the kale in the strainer with the lemon zest and juice. Lots of lemon makes this good!

Toast the bread until brown and crispy, about 3 minutes. Spread the toast thickly with hummus. Set aside two pieces to top the sandwiches. On the remaining two pieces, sprinkle the green onions, pile cilantro on top, and then lay a few slices of lemon on the cilantro. Place a large handful of lemon-filled kale on top of each sandwich half and top with the other two toast slices.

Variation:

Add a thick slice of tomato to each sandwich.

E2 Wraps and Pitas

These recipes will take advantage of all the great leftovers from your previous dinners. Our vehicle for delivering these glorious leftovers is a wrap, a pita, a tortilla, or a big old leafy green!

E2 Basics Pita

Up the street from the station there used to be a restaurant called The Pita Pit, which had a wild method of slicing open the top quarter of the pita and then peeling it back. Then they stuffed in all the ingredients, took the top, folded it down over the filling, and rolled the whole thing up. It's a simple and easy technique, and makes a no-nonsense wrap.

If you can't get your pita to roll up perfectly, don't get frustrated: This technique requires a thin, large, and pliable pita.

If you have a gluten allergy, try large corn tortillas or wheat-free wraps.

Serves 2

2 pieces whole grain pita
Leftovers from dinner
Romaine lettuce, chopped
Balsamic vinegar to taste

Warm the pitas in a skillet or microwave to make them pliable. Open the top quarter of each pita and stuff with leftovers and romaine lettuce. Lightly drizzle the pita filling with balsamic vinegar. Fold up the top portion and eat as is, or try to roll it up like a sleeping bag.

Variations:

Spread the inside of the pita with your choice of E2 spread or dip instead of dinner extras. Toss in your favorite fresh vegetables. Season with fresh lime or lemon juice in place of balsamic vinegar.

E2 Basics Wrap

This is an old standby for those times when you open up the refrigerator door and don't know what to eat.

Serves 2

2 large whole grain wraps
Healthy Homemade Hummus (see page 236)
1 tomato, sliced
1 cup shredded romaine lettuce
Cracked pepper to taste

Toast wraps in a skillet or directly over a gas flame. Spread each wrap thickly with hummus. Layer with tomatoes and top with lettuce. Season with pepper, and roll into a burrito.

Variations:

Use your choice of E2 spread or dip in place of hummus. Use spinach instead of romaine, then bake in the oven at 450°F for 10 minutes.

Rip's Big Leaf Special

This is a variation on the green leafy wrap. I wanted to take it to the next level and created this great little number.

Serves 2

2 large whole collard green leaves
Healthy Homemade Hummus with jalapeño (see page 236)
1 roasted red bell pepper, sliced into strips (see Roasting Peppers and
    Fresh Chilies, page 139)
1 cup corn
2 green onions, chopped
2 roma tomatoes, chopped
1 cup cooked brown rice (see E2 Brown Rice, page 175)

Blanch the leaves in a saucepan filled with a half-inch of boiling water for 2 minutes. Spread the leaves with hummus. Layer on the remaining ingredients, and roll into a burrito.

Green Leafy Wrap

This terrific wrap will alter your perception of reality, or at least lunch. It's great for anyone who wants to lose weight fast while taking in a huge dose of nutrients. You'll be amazed at how great the ingredients taste when the bread doesn't get in the way.

Serves 2

2 large whole collard green leaves
Healthy Homemade Hummus (see page 236)
1 tomato, sliced
1 cup shredded romaine lettuce
Cracked pepper to taste

Blanch the collard greens in a saucepan filled with a half inch of boiling water for 2 minutes, which makes the leaves easy to work with and brings out their magnificent deep green color. Spread leaves thickly with hummus. Layer with tomato and top with lettuce. Season with pepper, and roll into a burrito.

Variations:

Use the leaves unblanched.

Use your choice of E2 spread or dip in place of hummus.

Use romaine lettuce (unblanched) or Swiss chard leaves in place of collard greens.

Add cucumber and carrots, thinly sliced lengthwise.

For outrageously healthy hors d'oeuvres, cut wraps into 2-inch pieces and stab with a toothpick.

E2 Almighty Healthy Wrap

Our very own Station 2 won the 2003 Austin Fire Department's Healthy Wagon Contest with this very healthful and tasty lunch/dinner wrap. The judges included three experts—the Fire Department's in-house health specialist, a local representative from the American Heart Association, and a member of the Mayor's Council for Physical Fitness.

The department also sponsored an awards presentation at which we received a little red wagon, a healthy low-fat cookbook, a salad spinner, and fifty dollars to use for a future healthy wagon.

This wrap also makes an excellent dinner.

Serves 2

1 onion, chopped
1 bell pepper, seeded and chopped
½ cup sliced mushrooms
1 cup corn kernels, rinsed and drained
Healthy Homemade Hummus with roasted red bell pepper (see page 236)
2 large whole grain wraps
1½ cups black beans, rinsed and drained
1 roasted poblano pepper, cut into strips (see Roasting Peppers and Fresh Chilies, page 139)

2 cups fresh spinach
Guacamole (see page 238)
Salsa (see page 240)

Preheat the oven to 450°F. In a large skillet on medium-high heat, sauté the onion with a little bit of water until translucent, about 5 minutes. Add the bell pepper and cook for 2 to 3 minutes. Add the mushrooms and corn for another 1 to 2 minutes.

Spread a layer of hummus on each wrap. Add the sautéed vegetables, beans, poblano strips, and fresh spinach. Roll into a burrito. Place the wraps on a baking sheet, seam side down, and bake for 8 to 10 minutes. Serve warm, and top with guacamole and salsa.

Variation:
Substitute one 4-ounce can of drained green chilies for the roasted poblano pepper.

E2 Lunch Salads

On the Engine 2 Diet, we eat as many raw and cooked vegetables as possible—particularly green leafy ones. At dinner I always have either a spinach or romaine lettuce salad or large servings of steamed or sautéed greens such as kale, collard greens, turnip greens, or mustard greens.

I want you to get into the habit of eating as many greens and salads as you can. Soon you will crave them as you used to crave cheese and/or sweets.

Lunch salads serve 2.

Baby Field Greens Salad
Greens, greens, greens! Greens are the king of all foods! All food originates from greens. Remember, even carnivores feast on animals who themselves are built from greens. So bypass the recycled greens and go straight to the mother lode.

½ small red onion, sliced into ¼-inch rounds
1 tablespoon molasses

1 pound package baby field greens
1 cup grated carrot
1 cup grapes
15-ounce can butter beans, rinsed and drained
6 walnuts in pieces
Cracked black pepper to taste
Dijon Dressing (see page 232)

Cook the onion in a skillet on high heat for 5 minutes, stirring frequently and occasionally adding a few drops of water. When the slices begin to brown, stir in the molasses and 1 tablespoon water. Stir for a minute longer, until the liquid is absorbed, then remove from the heat.

Place the baby field greens in a large bowl. Arrange the carrots, grapes, beans, walnuts, and caramelized onions on top of the greens. Season with cracked pepper. Dress lightly with the dressing, and toss the ingredients together.

E2 Basics Salad

Instead of using iceberg lettuce, which has a low nutrient value, use romaine. Incredibly robust, it's loaded with more than 40 percent protein and bursting with antioxidants, phytochemicals, and other micronutrients. Remember, no food is nutritionally superior to greens. None.

½ head romaine lettuce, rinsed and torn into bite-size pieces
11-ounce can mandarin oranges, drained
1 red bell pepper, seeded and sliced into strips
½ avocado, peeled and sliced
Cracked black pepper to taste
E2 Basics Dressing (see page 232)

Place the lettuce in a large bowl. Arrange fruit and vegetables atop the lettuce, and season with cracked pepper. Dress lightly with the dressing, and toss ingredients together.

Variation:
Add roasted red bell pepper strips.

Red Tip Lettuce Salad

When you're not in the mood for a robust romaine lettuce salad, a softer red tip lettuce is a nice alternative.

1 small head red tip lettuce, rinsed and sliced into ½-inch strips
½ cucumber with skin on, sliced into rounds
2 small tomatoes, sliced
1 mango, peeled and chopped
Cracked pepper to taste
Peanut Dressing (see page 233)

Place the lettuce in a large bowl. Arrange the cucumber, tomatoes, and mango on top of the lettuce. Season with cracked pepper. Dress lightly with the dressing, and toss the ingredients together.

Spring Greens Salad

More good news about greens: Ounce for ounce, they are the greatest source of protein on the planet. Surprised? What do you think gives the elephant, cow, ape, bull, and giraffe their muscle and size? Greens. This clever combination of ingredients will make you feel that it's the first day of spring whenever you smell them.

8 ounces spring greens
14-ounce can artichoke hearts, drained
1 green bell pepper, seeded and sliced into strips
1 apple, diced
Cracked pepper to taste
Orange Hummus Dressing (see page 234)

Place the greens in a large bowl. Arrange the vegetables and fruit on top of the greens. Season with cracked pepper. Dress lightly with the dressing, and toss the ingredients together.

Spinach Salad

Dark leafy greens are the holy grail of all foods. Never forget this as you forage forward on your E2 journey.

8 ounces baby spinach greens
½ small red onion, sliced thin
6 black or Kalamata olives
1 orange, peeled and segmented
Cracked pepper to taste
Sesame Seed Dressing (see page 233)

Place the spinach in a large bowl. Arrange the onion, olives, and orange segments on top of the spinach. Season with cracked pepper. Dress the salad lightly with the dressing, and toss the ingredients together.

Variation:
Add one 15-ounce can chickpeas, rinsed and drained.

E2 DINNERS

Breakfast is a snap, lunch is a jiff, but dinner is a horse of a different color. Dinner is when we all pull up our bootstraps (or at Engine 2, our suspenders) and work as a group to create a meal with a lot of variety, great taste, and beautiful presentation. Over the course of the six years we ate plant-strong, we found a certain stride and rhythm that made cooking at the firehouse a joyous, team-building activity.

E2 Brown Rice

There are many great ways to cook brown rice, which is an E2 staple. Here are four different recipes to suit your time frame, taste, and mood. The first method is unorthodox, but the payoff is a rice with a slightly nutty flavor that preserves the integrity of the individual grains. Allow about 45 minutes.

Makes about 5½ cups

2 cups uncooked short- or long-grain brown rice
3¾ cups hot water or low-sodium vegetable stock
2 tablespoons Bragg Liquid Aminos

Sauté the rice in a large skillet on high heat for 5 minutes, stirring constantly until the rice begins to brown and pop. Add the water or vegetable stock and Bragg's. Reduce the heat to medium, and cook uncovered for another 25 minutes or until the liquid has been absorbed and only a few bubbles of water show between the grains of rice. Turn off the heat, cover, and let the rice sit on a warm stove for 10 minutes.

If the rice has achieved the desired consistency but some liquid remains, cook on high uncovered until the liquid is gone. If the liquid has been absorbed but some rice sticks to the bottom of the pan, add ⅛ cup hot water, cover, and let sit for 5 minutes. Fluff the rice with a fork, and leave uncovered until ready to serve. Allow the rice to cool completely before refrigerating.

The second method is the traditional method of using a saucepan with two parts water to one part rice. Allow about 50 minutes.

2 cups water or low-sodium vegetable stock
1 cup uncooked short- or long-grain brown rice

In a medium saucepan bring 2 cups of water or stock to a boil. Add the rice and wait for the water to come to a boil again. Turn the heat down to a simmer, cover, and cook for 45 minutes. Remove from heat and let stand for 5 minutes before serving.

The third method is the easiest and produces a perfect rice every time—the rice cooker. For those of you who are always on the go, a rice cooker is a must-have item on the E2 Diet. Turn it on and walk away. Allow 30 minutes.

1 cup uncooked short- or long-grain brown rice
1¼ cups water or low-sodium vegetable stock

Place rice and water or stock into the rice cooker and push the start button. The rice cooker will automatically turn off when the rice is done. Dig in!

Finally, for those of you who have zero time in your day, there is now a precooked brown rice in most freezer sections. Whole Foods makes a 365 brand precooked brown rice that can be ready lickety-split. Allow 3 minutes in a microwave and 6 minutes on a stove top.

In Microwave:

Put desired amount of 365 brand rice in a microwave-safe dish. Cook on high for 1½ to 2 minutes per cup of rice. Let stand for 1 minute. Remove and serve.

On Stove Top:

To maintain moisture while heating, add 1 to 2 tablespoons water and keep covered. Heat rice on medium-low heat in a saucepan or skillet. Stir frequently until heated through (5 to 7 minutes per cup of rice).

E2 Dinner Plates

An E2 dinner plate is a meal of plant-savvy foods that complement each other well in taste, texture, and presentation.

Dinner plates were a big hit during the original Engine 2 Pilot Study, in which we offered fourteen different combinations. Here are five that complement each other wonderfully.

They also make great leftovers when placed in a green leafy wrap, toasted pita, or corn tortilla.

E2 Black Beans and Rice

This is a mainstay dinner dish that is as basic as they come and, oh, so good. Just like my morning bowl of cereal, I've been eating this meal for more than three decades. This is also a great meal to serve when you're having extra guests over for dinner.

Serve with healthy chips or warm corn tortillas.

Serves 3 to 4

2 (15-ounce) cans black beans, rinsed and drained
1 to 1½ cups water or low-sodium vegetable stock
1 tablespoon Bragg Liquid Aminos
1 teaspoon chili powder

2 or 3 tomatoes, chopped
1 bunch green onions, chopped
8-ounce can water chestnuts, drained
1 cup corn, fresh, frozen, or canned
2 bell peppers, seeded and chopped
1 bunch cilantro, rinsed and chopped
1 avocado, peeled and sliced
3 cups cooked brown rice (see E2 Brown Rice, page 175)
Salsa (see page 240) or low-sodium tamari to taste

Heat the beans in a saucepan with the water or stock, Bragg's, and chili powder. Place the vegetables, cilantro, and avocado in individual bowls. To serve, place several big spoonfuls of brown rice onto large plates and ladle beans on top. Add generous handfuls of the vegetables, cilantro, and avocado on top of the beans. Top with salsa or tamari.

Variations:
Drizzle with E2 Sour Cream (see page 239).
Use pinto or kidney beans in place of black beans.

Red Beans over Quinoa with Kale

For our honeymoon, Jill and I hiked the Inca Trail to Machu Picchu, the religious citadel of the Incan Empire. During the four-day excursion, hikers are required to hire porters, a guide, and a cook. We requested plant-strong meals for breakfast, lunch, and dinner, and our helpers ably rose to the occasion.

Our guide, Fisher, told us about the holy grain that the Incan warriors used for stamina and strength—quinoa, which is a cousin to green leafy vegetables and wonderfully high in protein. We had this for dinner one night with red beans and greens and it put a kick in our step the next day. Serve the quinoa, beans, and kale nestled side by side on large dinner plates.

Serves 2 to 4

5 cups water
2 cups quinoa, rinsed

1 onion, chopped
2 bay leaves
1 clove garlic, minced
2 green bell peppers, seeded and chopped
1 teaspoon dried thyme
1 tablespoon cider vinegar
2 (15-ounce) cans kidney beans, rinsed and drained
1 bunch kale, rinsed and coarsely chopped (see Preparing Leafy Greens
    on page 140)

For Quinoa:

In a large saucepan, bring 3¾ cups of the water to a boil. Add the rinsed quinoa, stir once, and cover. Cook on medium heat for 25 minutes. If any water remains, cook uncovered for a few minutes longer. The quinoa should not be soggy. Remove from heat and let the quinoa sit covered for 10 minutes. Fluff gently with a fork.

For Kidney Beans:

Sauté the onion and bay leaves on medium heat in a saucepan for 5 minutes until the onions are translucent. If the onions start to stick, add a few drops of water and stir. Add the garlic and bell pepper and cook for 5 minutes, until the peppers soften. Add the thyme, vinegar, kidney beans, and 1 cup of water, and cook on low heat for 5 minutes, until the broth thickens. You can speed this process by mashing the beans a few times with a potato masher.

For Kale:

Place the kale with the remaining ¼ cup of water in a large pot on medium heat and cover. Cook the greens for 3 to 5 minutes, stirring occasionally, until they are wilted and tender.

Rip's Tip

To rinse quinoa, use a coffee filter or handheld mesh strainer with small holes because the grains are very small.

E2 POP QUIZ

Q: Which has more cholesterol, a 3-ounce piece of red meat, or a 3-ounce piece of chicken breast, or a 3-ounce piece of tuna?

A: The red meat, chicken, and fish all have the same amount of cholesterol—80 milligrams.

Tofu Steaks and Mushrooms with Mashed Potatoes and Green Beans

These steaks have all the taste and texture you'd expect from a five-star steakhouse restaurant, but you won't have a food hangover the next morning, nor will you be doing any permanent damage to your arteries. Serve tofu steaks and vegetables side by side on large dinner plates.

Serves 2 to 3

1 pound extra-firm tofu, drained and cut into 6 slices
8 ounces mushrooms, sliced
1 tablespoon low-sodium soy sauce
Cracked pepper to taste
1 cup arugula or baby spinach
2 green onions, sliced thin
10 small red potatoes, scrubbed and cut in half
½ cup unsweetened plant-based milk
1 tablespoon fresh rosemary, chopped
2 (16-ounce) cans green beans (or 1 pound frozen or fresh)
⅛ cup water
1 tablespoon Bragg Liquid Aminos
2 tablespoons home-toasted sesame seeds (see Toasting Nuts and Seeds, page 139)

For Tofu and Mushrooms:

Press the tofu with a kitchen towel to remove excess water. Place the tofu and mushrooms in a large skillet. Season with soy sauce and pepper. Cook together on medium heat for 10 minutes, turning the tofu once to ensure even browning. Place the cooked steaks and mushrooms over a handful of fresh arugula on a dinner plate. Sprinkle the steaks with green onions. Reserve the skillet for the green beans.

For Mashed Potatoes:

Steam the potatoes for 10 minutes, until tender. Place in a large bowl and mash with the plant-based milk, rosemary, and pepper.

For Green Beans:

Cook the beans on medium heat in a covered skillet with the water for 4 minutes or until tender and bright green in color. Season with Bragg's. Sprinkle with sesame seeds.

Rip's Tip

Double the tofu recipe and save the extra for future tacos, salads, and quick snacks.

Roasted Bell Peppers, Baked Sweet Potatoes, and Galloping Greens with Cashew Sauce

This dinner plate is bursting with so much color (and so many antioxidants), you'll think you've been jettisoned into a rainbow. The strong, salty flavor of mustard greens is deliciously paired with the buttery sweetness of sweet potatoes.

I love roasting bell peppers. My favorite method is using a gas burner cranked up to high and turning the peppers with tongs. When the pepper is completely blackened, immediately place it under cold water and, using your fingers, peel off the black outer skin until a glistening, slick underbelly reveals itself.

Spruce up the galloping greens with a cashew or walnut tamari sauce. Both are Engine 2 favorites. Derick loves these sauces so much he's been caught putting them on his breakfast cereal.

Serve the vegetables side by side on large dinner plates.

Serves 2 to 3

2 large sweet potatoes, scrubbed and pricked with a fork
3 red, orange, or yellow bell peppers
1 pound package or bunch fresh mustard greens, rinsed and coarsely chopped
¼ cup water or orange juice
½ cup home-toasted cashews (see Toasting Nuts and Seeds, page 139)
1 tablespoon low-sodium tamari
2 cloves garlic

For Sweet Potatoes:

Preheat the oven to 450°F. Place the potatoes in a casserole dish and bake for 45 minutes, until they indent easily with finger pressure. Set aside to cool. Slice in half and serve with the skins on.

For Bell Peppers:

If you don't have a gas burner: Halve the peppers and remove the seeds. Place the halves cut-side down on a baking sheet. Cook on the oven rack above the sweet potatoes for 5 minutes, until the skins begin to bubble and blacken. Remove from the oven and allow to cool. Under running water, peel away the skins. Slice the flesh into 1-inch strips.

If you have a gas burner: Place the pepper directly on top of the burner, turn to high heat, and turn the pepper until it's completely blackened. This is best done with a long pair of tongs. Once the pepper is cool enough, peel, remove the seeds, and slice into 1-inch strips.

For Galloping Greens with Cashew Sauce:

Place the mustard greens and water in a large pot over medium heat and cover. Cook for 4 to 6 minutes, stirring occasionally, until the greens are wilted and tender. In a blender, process the cashews, tamari, and garlic, adding a small amount of water as necessary to combine. Keep adding water until the mixture has the consistency of a smoothie. Spoon the cashew sauce over the cooked greens.

Rip's Tip

Cashews and walnuts are generally interchangeable, especially in sauces, so if you prefer walnuts, use them.

Cravotta's Couscous with Tomatoes and Asparagus

This couscous recipe was the invention of Engine 2 Diet participant Mark Cravotta, an ingenious interior designer with an impeccable eye for mixing and matching colors in a house—and on a dinner plate. As in any well-designed creation, the flavors of these various ingredients blend together beautifully.

To serve, place a generous spoonful of couscous in the center of a dinner plate and top with a broiled tomato. Place asparagus around the couscous, just as Mark does.

Serves 3 to 4

1¾ cups water or low-sodium vegetable stock
2 cups whole wheat couscous
4 to 6 tablespoons molasses
6 to 8 dried apricots, diced
½ cup pecans, chopped
4 medium tomatoes
Cracked pepper to taste
Drizzle of balsamic vinegar
1 pound asparagus
Tabasco sauce (optional)

For Couscous:

In a medium saucepan, bring the water or vegetable stock to a boil. Turn off the heat and stir in the couscous. Cover and let sit for 10 minutes. Meanwhile, heat up the molasses in a separate small saucepan. Add the molasses, apricots, and pecans to the couscous. Fluff gently with a fork.

For Tomatoes:

Preheat the oven to 450°F. Cut the cores from the tomatoes and place them upright in a casserole dish. Season with pepper. Drizzle balsamic vinegar into the core. Bake for 20 minutes or until the skins are peeling away and the tomatoes are softening.

For Asparagus:

Snap the woody ends from the asparagus. Place the spears in a skillet on high heat and season with pepper. Cook for 4 to 6 minutes stirring occasionally or until the spears begin to brown slightly. If you wish, add some Tabasco sauce.

Variations:

Asparagus is also excellent steamed or lightly sautéed.

If you don't like asparagus, you can sauté 1 pound of frozen artichoke hearts in a saucepan with the juice of 1 lemon and cracked pepper, and add to the dinner plate.

E2 Burgers

Let's face it. Burgers are easy, they're all-American, and everyone loves 'em, whether you're flipping them on the grill for a Fourth of July barbecue, pan-frying them in a skillet for a midweek dinner, roasting them in the oven for a weekend supper, or microwaving one for a quick lunch. I've included a wide variety of veggie burgers to suit your fancy.

E2 EZ Burgers

Healthy burger substitutes abound in the frozen section of most supermarkets. We have four delicious varieties of plant-strong burgers available at Whole Foods Market. Look for the Engine 2 Plant-Strong Burgers: Italian Fennel, Pinto Habanero, Poblano Black Bean, and Tuscan Kale White Bean in the freezer section. These can be broiled on a parchment-lined baking sheet, cooked on a stove top in a skillet, browned on a grill, or thrown in a microwave by following the instructions on the box. Serve on toasted whole grain buns with lots of fresh toppings, healthy condiments, and your choice of potato sides.

Serves 4

4 thawed Engine 2 Plant-Strong burgers

Low-sodium tamari or Bragg Liquid Aminos

Cracked pepper to taste

4 whole grain buns

Healthy condiments (see E2-Approved Foods to Keep in Your Pantry, page 127)

Lettuce, tomato slices, onion slices, dill pickles, or other favorite burger toppings

Sprinkle the patties lightly with tamari and season with pepper. Brown the patties in a skillet with a few drops of water on high for 3 minutes on each side, until brown. Remove the burgers from the skillet but leave the skillet on the heat. Cut the buns in half and toast in the hot skillet. Assemble the burgers with your favorite fixings.

Variations:

In the hot skillet, on the grill, or in the broiler, cook onions, red bell peppers, and/or mushrooms and add them to the burgers. Top with avocado slices, Guacamole (see page 238), Three-Bean Chili (see page 220), or canned jalapeño slices.

Monica Cravotta, 35

Public Relations Consultant

I think it's tougher for guys to do this than for women. It's considered masculine to eat steak, not broccoli. But I want to know, what is more masculine—eating a slab of meat, or to be around healthy to take care of your wife and kids? Which would you choose? I'd like to think that most men would choose the family.

New York Times Veggie Burgers

When the *New York Times* photographer came to our firehouse to take our picture, we were making these veggie burgers for the first time. We used old-fashioned oats instead of quick oats and the result was a patty that did not want to hold together. We were able to squeeze them together for the photo, but we highly recommend the quick oats rather than the old-fashioned kind. Make extra for lunch the next day.

Makes about 8 patties

15-ounce can black beans, rinsed and drained
10-ounce can tomatoes with zesty mild chilies, drained
1 clove garlic, minced or pressed, or 1 teaspoon garlic powder
1 teaspoon onion powder
2 green onions, chopped
1 cup chopped carrots
1 cup chopped parsley or cilantro
2 cups quick rolled oats
8 whole grain buns
Fresh veggie toppings and healthy condiments

Preheat the oven to 450°F. Process the beans, tomatoes, garlic, onion powder, green onions, and carrots, using blender or food processor. Transfer the mixture to a large bowl and stir in the oats. Form into patties, place on a parchment-lined baking sheet, and bake for 8 minutes. Turn the oven up to broil and cook for 2 more minutes, until the tops are nicely browned. Toast the buns and pile on your favorite toppings.

Variation:

Sauté the burgers on medium heat in a skillet with a few drops of water for 5 minutes on each side, until both sides are browned.

Portobello Mushroom Burgers

Portobello mushroom burgers are healthy, hearty, juicy, and meaty-flavored—well suited for roasting or grilling. The black gills on the mushroom's underside hold in the flavor of a marinade or barbecue sauce superbly. Serve with healthy fries.

Makes 4 burgers

4 Portobello mushrooms, rinsed
Low-sodium tamari
Vegetarian Worcestershire sauce
Splash of beer (optional)
Cracked pepper to taste
1 large red onion, sliced into thin rounds
4 whole grain buns, toasted
Dijon mustard or Healthy Homemade Hummus (see page 236)
Tomato slices, lettuce, spinach, or other favorite burger toppings

Preheat the oven to 450°F. Snap the stems off the mushrooms and place the caps gill-side up on a parchment-lined baking sheet. Splash a few drops of tamari and Worcestershire (beer splash is optional) into each cap. Season with pepper. Trim the stems and place them in the caps. Cook on the baking sheet for 10 to 15 minutes, until the mushrooms are soft and filled with liquid. Enjoy the stems as starters!

While the mushrooms are roasting, cook the onion rounds on high heat in a skillet with a few drops of water for 5 minutes, stirring often, until wilted and brown.

Spread the buns with Dijon mustard or hummus. Place each mushroom on a toasted bun with cooked onion and your favorite fixings.

Variation:

Shake some barbecue sauce into the mushrooms instead of the tamari.

Sloppy Joes

Sloppy Joe sandwiches are well named—they're very, very messy. When was the last time you got to lick your fingers and slurp up the drippings off the plate? These are especially delicious with a side of steamed spinach and potato wedges.

Serves 4

1 onion, chopped
2 cups cooked red lentils
½ cup water
6 ounces tomato paste
1 teaspoon low-sodium tamari
1 teaspoon vegetarian Worcestershire sauce
1 teaspoon brown sugar
4 whole grain buns, toasted
1 onion, sliced into thin rounds (optional)
Sliced dill pickles

Sauté the onion on high heat in a skillet with a few drops of water for 3 minutes, until just translucent. Add the cooked lentils and ¼ cup of the water to the skillet and cook for 5 minutes, until warmed through. Stir in the tomato paste. Add the remaining ¼ cup water and stir until thoroughly mixed, using more water as necessary to make a thick sauce. Stir in the tamari, Worcestershire, and sugar. Place a generous amount of filling into each bun. Top with sliced onion, if using, and pickles.

Candle Café Brown Rice and Lentil Burgers

Near the end of a shift in early 2007, we heard a knock at the fire station's front door. Steve, Derick, and I opened it to find a group of people who asked if we were "the world-famous vegan firefighters."

Proudly, we said we were. One of the women then looked us over for several seconds and exclaimed, "Wow! Veganism never looked so good!"

Steve and I are six feet, two inches tall, while Derick is six feet, four inches.

The visitors included a couple named Bart and Joy, who told us that they were from New York City, where they owned and managed two renowned vegan restaurants, the Candle Café and Candle 79. Bart and Joy had won the New York lottery several years back and used the money to help start their restaurants. Now they were on a reconnaissance trip to investigate opening up a vegan restaurant in Austin.

Before they left, they presented us with a signed copy of *The Candle Café Cookbook*. And so, in honor of Bart and Joy, here's a brown rice and lentil burger recipe adapted from their book.

Makes about 8 patties

3½ cups water
½ cup uncooked French lentils, rinsed and drained
1 cup uncooked brown rice
2 cloves garlic, chopped
1 medium red onion, chopped
2 red bell peppers, seeded and diced
1 teaspoon sea salt
1 teaspoon chili powder
Whole grain flour
8 whole grain buns

Preheat the oven to 350°F. In a medium saucepan, bring 1½ cups of the water to a boil. Add the lentils, reduce the heat to low, and cook until the beans are softened, about 15 minutes. Drain and set aside. Meanwhile, in another medium saucepan, bring the remaining 2 cups of water to a boil, add the rice, reduce the heat to low, cover, and simmer until the rice is just tender, about 40 minutes. Drain and set aside.

While the rice is cooking, sauté the garlic, onion, and peppers in a skillet with a few drops of water for about 5 minutes, until lightly browned.

In a large bowl, combine the lentils, rice, and vegetables. Add the salt and chili powder and mix well. Add a bit of flour to hold the mixture together, if needed. Form into burger-sized patties and place on a baking sheet. Bake the burgers until slightly firm, about 15 minutes. Serve on warmed buns.

E2 Potato Sides

A burger just wouldn't be complete without a potato side. I've included four different ways of preparing potatoes, depending on which burger you're craving and which potato calls out to you. Serve potatoes with E2 Burgers and a side of healthy ketchup. Make extra potato sides for use in wraps, pitas, and Tex-Mex tacos.

Sweet Potato Fries

We loved sweet potato fries at Station 2. Nothing could be easier. We left the skin on for maximum nutrients and flavor. Sweet potatoes with their golden orange color are a rich and vibrant source of beta-carotene—hence the bold, carrot-like color.

2 sweet potatoes with skins on, scrubbed and sliced into ¼–½ inch strips

Preheat the oven to 450°F. Place the potato slices on a parchment-lined baking sheet and cover with aluminum foil. Cook for 20 minutes, then remove the foil and flip the fries over with a spatula. Return the sheet to the oven and cook uncovered for another 10 to 20 minutes to allow the slices to brown.

Rip's Tip

The thinner your slices, the faster they cook. They are most delicious when light brown—but take care not to burn them.

Potato Wedges

You should be able to find some healthy potato wedges in the freezer section of your grocery store. Every once in a while, treat yourself to the ease of cutting open a bag, throwing the pieces on a cookie sheet, and baking until crispy. If you can't find healthy frozen potato wedges, use fresh baking potatoes.

16 ounces frozen potato wedges or sliced fresh potatoes

Preheat the oven to 450°F. Place the potatoes on a parchment-lined baking sheet and cover with aluminum foil. Cook for 15 minutes, then remove the foil and flip the slices over with a spatula. Return the sheet to the oven and cook uncovered for another 5 to 10 minutes to allow the slices to brown.

Sweet Potato Rounds

This is a slight variation on the sliced sweet potato fries. Here you'll be cutting them so they are like thick potato chips. They'll cook faster and have a slightly different taste and texture. Just as the shape and texture of a pasta can do wonders for changing up a pasta dish, the same is true with cutting up your potatoes.

2 sweet potatoes with skins on, scrubbed and sliced into ½-inch rounds (thinner if you like)

Preheat the oven to 450°F. Place the rounds on a parchment-lined baking sheet and cover with aluminum foil. Cook for 15 minutes, then remove the foil and flip the slices over with a spatula. Return the sheet to the oven and cook uncovered for another 10 minutes to allow the slices to brown.

Steamed Red Potatoes

These little buggers are cute as buttons and, when steamed, are as smooth and creamy as freshly made peanut butter. Make a whole bunch and eat some the next day as a snack dipped in an E2 spread such as Healthy Homemade Hummus (see page 236). They're great cold and travel well.

1 pound small red potatoes

Scrub the potatoes. If they are bigger than a golf ball, cut them in half. Steam for 10 to 15 minutes, or until a fork glides through the potato with ease.

Variation:

Slice the potatoes in half and place on a parchment-lined backing sheet in the broiler until the tops of the potatoes start to brown and bubble up, about 10 to 14 minutes.

E2 Pasta

At Engine 2, we loved pasta any way we could get it: spaghetti, angel hair, fettuccine, linguine, gnocchi, penne, elbows, and macaroni. However, our one demand was that it must be a whole grain pasta rather than a white one or a blend. Filled with fiber and complex carbohydrates, a whole grain pasta meal was always a regular occurrence at our station.

Begin every pasta meal with a starter salad!

Put kale or any fresh greens in the water with the pasta a few minutes before the pasta is ready. Also, nutritional yeast or finely ground raw cashews make great substitutes for Parmesan cheese.

Gnocchi and Red Sauce

These little potato-filled monsters go down way too easily for something that is so difficult to pronounce (*nyo-kee*). Boil them in water, and when they float to the surface—usually within 4 minutes—they're done. An easy way to get greens, such as kale or Swiss chard, into your meal is to add them to the water and bring them out with the gnocchi.

Serves 3 to 4

2 (24-ounce) jars pasta sauce (see E2-Approved Foods to Keep in Your Pantry, page 127)
½ cup cooked white beans
2 (2-pound) packages whole grain gnocchi

Combine the pasta sauce and white beans in a large saucepan on medium heat. Simmer until warm. Bring a large pot of water to a boil. Add the gnocchi and cook until they float to the surface, about 4 minutes, then drain. Spoon the sauce over the gnocchi.

Variations:

Add sautéed onion and mushrooms, fresh garlic, oregano, rosemary, basil, or a splash of red wine to the sauce.

Mushroom Stroganoff

One night while watching the Food Network at the firehouse, we saw television chef Rachael Ray make a mushroom sauce with three types of mushrooms, shallots, fresh thyme, broth, and milk. She also sautéed several chicken breasts that she sliced and added to the mushrooms. This entree went over a heaping platter of orzo (rice-shaped pasta).

Rachael then served a romaine lettuce salad with a dressing that called for a half gallon of olive oil, which is considerably more than anyone should use.

Rachael also emphasized feeding your soul as well as your stomach, and that taking the time to make a homemade meal is always well worth the effort. On that point we heartily agree. So here we offer a plant-strong version of Rachael's dish: a fabulous mushroom sauce over healthy noodles.

Serves 3 to 4

1 large yellow onion, chopped
1 cup sliced cremini or other wild mushrooms
1 cup sliced white mushrooms
4 cloves garlic, minced
3 tablespoons whole wheat flour
1 tablespoon balsamic vinegar
½ cup unsweetened plant-based milk
Ground thyme to taste
16 ounces whole grain fettuccini noodles, cooked

Cook the onion in a skillet with a little water on high heat for 3 minutes. Add the mushrooms and garlic, then cook until the mushrooms begin to release their juices, about 5 minutes. In a saucepan over medium heat, combine the flour, vinegar, and plant-based milk. Stir vigorously with a whisk until the sauce thickens and the flour evenly dissolves. Add the thyme. Serve warm over the cooked noodles.

Pasta Primavera

"Worming," something found in all firehouses, means pulling a practical joke on an individual or group (the term evokes a worm burrowing down and getting under the skin). Besides being fun, it serves a valuable purpose, giving you an excellent sense of someone's true colors in the face of chaos and confusion. Many wonderful and creative worms have been inflicted by firefighters on other firefighters over the years. Here's one that Engine 4 once pulled on Engine 2 while we were out checking hydrants: When we returned to the station, we found all of our toilet paper gone, flour on top of every blade of every ceiling fan, mattresses and box springs interchanged on our beds, sugar placed in the mop bucket, and of course, since we were the plant-healthy fire station, beef bouillon cubes strategically inserted inside each showerhead.

This pasta dish has no bouillon, or any other meat, in it. It's colorful, hearty, tasty, and a great way to get greens into your evening meal. It also makes for wonderful leftovers. We used to make a tub full and polish it off before going home the next day at noon.

Serves 3 to 4

1 red onion, chopped
1 clove garlic, minced
15-ounce can corn, rinsed and drained
1 jalapeño pepper, minced (remove the ribs and seeds to reduce heat)
1 green or red bell pepper, seeded and chopped
1 bunch fresh kale, rinsed and chopped (see Preparing Leafy Greens on page 140)
14.5-ounce can diced tomatoes with juice
24-ounce jar pasta sauce (see E2-Approved Foods to Keep in Your Pantry, page 127)
16 ounces whole grain spaghetti, cooked
½ cup raw cashews, finely ground

Sauté the onion, garlic, and corn with a few drops of water in a large skillet on medium heat for 5 minutes. Add the jalapeño, bell pepper, and kale to the skillet and cook for 3 minutes. Add the diced tomatoes and pasta sauce to the vegetables. Ladle the sauce over the pasta and top with the cashews.

Linguine and Creamy Alfredo Sauce

Because it's nice to have options other than red sauce, I've included this recipe we've been perfecting. The cashew nuts supply some fat and add texture and allow the sauce to stick to each noodle, while the other ingredients enhance the taste.

Serves 3 to 4

12-ounces Mori-Nu silken tofu
2 cups unsweetened plant-based milk
¼ cup nutritional yeast flakes
¼ cup soaked raw cashews (soak 1 hour)
1 tablespoon onion powder
¾ teaspoon sea salt
½ teaspoon garlic powder
½ teaspoon white pepper
1 white onion, diced
1 tablespoon fresh parsley, chopped
1 tablespoon fresh thyme, chopped
1 tablespoon fresh basil, chopped
¼ cup water
¼ cup white wine
¼ cup whole wheat flour
16 ounces whole grain linguine, cooked

Blend all the ingredients from the tofu to the pepper until smooth. Sauté the onion with the herbs and water in a saucepan over medium heat until the onions are translucent and all the liquid has evaporated. Be careful not to brown the onion during this step. Pour in the wine, swirling it around in the pan to absorb the heat until it begins to sizzle. Add the blended ingredients to the wine and onions, continuously whisking the sauce.

When a gentle bubbling starts, gradually add the flour and continue to whisk until the sauce has thickened. Remove from heat. The sauce will be frothy at this point. Continue whisking for 1 minute, or until the sauce has settled and is smooth and thick. Ladle over the pasta.

Variation:
Add artichoke hearts and mushrooms to the sauce.

Bow Ties with Pesto

Bow ties with pesto are a nice deviation from other pasta dishes. They make a great dinner and go beautifully with black beans, roasted bell peppers, and asparagus.

This dish is good the next day as a cold salad mixed with lettuce, fresh vegetables, and beans.

Serves 3 to 4

3 cloves garlic
1 cup home-toasted walnuts (see Toasting Nuts and Seeds, page 139)
3 bunches or 2 packed cups fresh basil
½ cup unsweetened plant-based milk or water to process
16 ounces whole grain bow ties, cooked

Blend the garlic and nuts briefly in a food processor. Add the basil and plant-based milk, and process to a thick consistency. Toss well with the pasta.

E2 Pizza

While Engine 2 was working at a public educational event at the annual University of Texas fair day, more than one thousand kids climbed into the engine in groups of four and five to hear us give a short talk on fire safety.

As the kids were leaving, I asked them to tell me their favorite food. The number one answer: "Pizza!"

Well, we love pizza, too. But ours is always on a whole grain crust and overflows with vegetables—and no cheese.

For a quick and easy meal, buy the Engine 2 Plant-Strong pizza crusts or Nature's Hilights crusts in the frozen section. Also, you can use large pita breads in a pinch. And always personalize your pizza with your favorite toppings.

Supreme Pizza

The mother of one of my good friends always used to exclaim how leftover pizza, warm or cold, was "absolutely divine." That reminds me of a pizza joke. Q: How are sex and pizza the same? A: When it's good, it's really good, and when it's bad, it's still pretty darn good.

    This pizza has the potential to get out of control so use caution!

Serves 2 to 3

24-ounce jar pizza sauce (see E2-Approved Foods to Keep in Your Pantry, page 127)
2 whole grain pizza crusts
1 cup thawed, rinsed, and drained frozen spinach
1 cup sliced mushrooms1 onion, sliced thin
2 cloves garlic, minced
2 red bell peppers, seeded and sliced
2 veggie burger patties, thawed and chopped
½ cup olives, sliced
4 roma tomatoes, sliced
1 to 2 tablespoons nutritional yeast

    Preheat the oven to 425°F. Spread a thick layer of sauce on the crusts. Cover with a generous amount of spinach and top with the remaining ingredients except for the yeast. Cook on a parchment-lined baking sheet or pizza stone for 15 to 20 minutes. Sprinkle the pizzas with nutritional yeast before serving.

Green Pizza

Before the Esselstyn family embarked on a plant-powered diet, we ate just about anything and everything—and my mother, Ann, and I were always able to devour more than anyone else. One night at a pizza parlor in upstate New York, we had a family pizza-eating contest that came down to my mother and me. We tied at eleven pieces each, all dripping with cheese, pepperoni, sausage, and ham.

This pizza is quite a departure—it's our lean, mean, and green pizza pie. We take all the rockin' green ingredients and place them together in this one band that'll be nutrient-packed music to your ears.

I bet Ann and I could eat *fifteen* pieces each of this delicacy!

Serves 2 to 3

24-ounce jar pasta sauce (see E2-Approved Foods to Keep in Your Pantry, page 127)
2 whole grain pizza crusts
½ cup thawed, rinsed, and drained frozen spinach
½ cup fresh whole basil leaves, packed
2 green bell peppers, seeded and diced
2 cups broccoli florets
½ cup sliced mushrooms
1 onion, diced
2 cloves garlic, minced
¼ cup finely ground raw cashews or 1 to 2 tablespoons nutritional yeast

Preheat the oven to 425°F. Generously spread the sauce on the crusts, and layer with the remaining ingredients except for the cashews. Top with the cashews or a sprinkling of nutritional yeast. Bake on a parchment-lined baking sheet or pizza stone for 15 minutes.

Rip's Tip

Nutritional yeast is a low-fat, low-sodium, deactivated yeast filled with vitamins, especially the B-complex ones. Often fortified with vitamin B12, it can take the place of cheese in many recipes, especially pizza.

Greek Pizza

Here we use our homemade Engine 2 pesto recipe (see Bow Ties with Pesto, page 196), then top the pizza with ingredients that are authentically Greek. After your first bite, stop and be still: Do you feel a warm ocean breeze on your face, sense a bit of sea salt in the air, and see the Parthenon in the distance?

Serves 2 to 3

1 cup Pesto (see Bow Ties with Pesto, page 196)
2 whole grain pizza crusts
1 red onion, sliced thin
4 roma tomatoes, sliced
½ cup Kalamata olives, chopped
14-ounce can artichoke hearts packed in water, drained

Preheat the oven to 425°F. Generously spread the sauce on the crusts, and layer with the remaining ingredients. Bake on a parchment-lined baking sheet or pizza stone for 15 minutes.

Bert's BBQ Pizza

Bert's Bar-B-Q was one of Austin's best joints of its kind and was located just two buildings down from our fire station. At 2:00 a.m. one morning, the 911 fire dispatcher received a call from a passerby reporting a great deal of smoke coming from the place. The dispatcher told him the cooks were probably just smoking some meat. Thirty minutes later another passerby called and reported some very serious smoke coming from Bert's. Again, the dispatcher wasn't too concerned until the caller said that he'd been barbecuing meat all his life and he had never seen anyone create this much smoke doing it.

So Engine 2 was dispatched to the fire—but it was too late. The building was destroyed. The next day several local radio deejays—jokingly—accused us firefighting plant-eaters of letting Bert's Bar-B-Q burn. But it just so happens we were not on duty that shift: the meat-eating, barbecue-loving B shifters were. So we were exonerated.

In a rather ironic twist, two weeks after Bert's burned down, one of Austin's best-known vegetarian restaurants, Mother's, also caught on fire. Once again, the deejays were wondering why the plant-eating firefighters didn't save the day. (As before, everything that could be done was done. And once again, it wasn't our shift.)

Barbecue is our simple twist on the supreme pizza. After slicing up the toppings, we place them in individual bowls on the kitchen counter. One at a time, each of us tops the crust, choosing the assortment and layout of ingredients he or she thinks will yield the most delicious and best-looking pizza. Presentation is always important!

Serves 2 to 3

6 ounces tomato paste
1 cup barbecue sauce
2 teaspoons dried oregano
2 whole grain pizza crusts
1 small red onion, sliced
1 red bell pepper, seeded and sliced
2 handfuls fresh spinach
20-ounce jar pineapple chunks in water, drained
½ cup finely ground cashews

Preheat the oven to 425°F. Mix the tomato paste, barbecue sauce, and oregano together in a bowl. Generously spread the sauce on the crusts, and layer with the vegetables and pineapple. Top with the cashews. Bake on a parchment-lined baking sheet or pizza stone for 15 minutes.

E2 Comfort Dinners

Among my fondest memories of my sister, Jane, and my brothers, Ted and Zeb, are the amazing trips we used to take to a ski slope about ten miles up the road from my grandparents' farm in upstate New York. We'd get there early and race up and down the mountain until they told us to go home. Then came the best part of the day: putting up the skis, sliding off our stiff boots, and sitting our exhausted bodies down in front of a roaring fire as we warmed our icy feet, drank hot chocolate, and ate one of Grandma Lil's scrumptious home-cooked dinners.

Let these comfort foods take you back in time to a similar place in your childhood.

E2 POP QUIZ

Q: What fruit has the highest percentage of protein?
A: A lemon, which is 16 percent protein.

Raise-the-Roof Sweet Potato–Vegetable Lasagna

I prepared this lasagna for my first cooking demonstration at the Whole Foods Culinary Center in Austin. Tim LaFuente, an award-winning chef who is also an Austin firefighter, asked me to join him at this event, where he made an angel hair pasta with chicken, bacon, butter, and oil.

Firefighters are naturally competitive, so the demonstration quickly turned into a contest. No one was declared the winner, but I walked away with my head high because the lasagna was a smashing success: another triumph for plant-happy cuisine!

This lasagna is so good Jill and I chose it to be the main dish at our wedding reception.

Serves 10 to 12

1 onion, chopped
1 small head of garlic, all cloves chopped or pressed
½ cup sliced mushrooms, sliced
1 head broccoli, chopped
2 carrots, chopped
2 red bell peppers, seeded and chopped
15-ounce can corn, rinsed and drained
12 ounces extra firm tofu
1 teaspoon dried oregano
1 teaspoon dried basil
1 teaspoon dried rosemary
½ teaspoon cayenne pepper
2 (24-ounce) jars pasta sauce (see E2-Approved Foods to Keep in Your Pantry, page 127)
2 boxes whole grain lasagna noodles
2 cups thawed, rinsed, and drained frozen spinach,
2 sweet potatoes, cooked and mashed
6 roma tomatoes, sliced thin
1 cup raw cashews, ground

Preheat the oven to 400°F. Sauté the onion and garlic with a few drops of water on high heat for 3 minutes in a wok or skillet. Add the mushrooms and cook until the onions are limp and the mushrooms give up their liquid, 2 to 3 minutes. Remove them to a large bowl with a slotted spoon. Reserve the mushroom liquid in the pan. Sauté the broccoli and carrots for 5 minutes and add to the mushroom bowl. Sauté the peppers and corn until just beginning to soften, about 2 minutes. Add them to the vegetable bowl. Drain the tofu by wrapping it in paper towels. Crumble it up directly in the towel and mix into the vegetable bowl. Add the herbs and cayenne to the vegetable bowl and combine.

To Assemble:

Cover the bottom of a 9-by-13-inch casserole dish with a layer of sauce. Add a layer of noodles. Cover the noodles with sauce. (This way the noodles cook in the oven, saving time and energy.) Spread the vegetable mixture over the sauced noodles. Cover with a layer of noodles and another dressing of sauce. Add the spinach to the second layer of sauced noodles. Cover the spinach with the mashed sweet potatoes. Add another layer of sauce, the final layer of noodles, and a last topping of sauce. Cover the lasagna with thinly sliced roma tomatoes.

Cover with foil and bake in the oven for 45 minutes. Remove the foil, sprinkle with the cashews, and return to the oven for 15 minutes. Let sit for 15 minutes before serving.

Lynn's Meatloaf

This is a great "meat" loaf recipe from one of the Engine 2 Pilot Study participants, Lynn Jocelyn. Lynn brought this to the Engine 2 potluck awards banquet and it disappeared before everyone could get a bite. She graciously brought two loaves over for Jill and me one week after Kole was born.

This meatloaf is wonderful the next day pan-fried on whole grain bread with mustard, pickles, and ketchup.

Serves 6

2 stalks celery, chopped
½ onion, chopped
2 cloves garlic, minced or pressed
10 ounces firm tofu, drained
¼ cup walnuts, finely ground
½ cup cooked brown lentils
1¼ cups quick-cooking oats
3 tablespoons low-sodium soy sauce
2 tablespoons ketchup (additional for topping)
1 tablespoon Dijon mustard
2 teaspoons dried parsley
½ teaspoon each dried thyme, sage, and rosemary

Preheat the oven to 375°F. Sauté the celery, onion, and garlic on high heat in a skillet with a few drops of water for 5 minutes, until tender. Remove from heat and cool. Mash the tofu in a large bowl. Stir in the cooked mixture and remaining ingredients, and combine well. Spoon the mixture into a parchment-lined loaf pan. Top with a layer of ketchup. Bake for 55 to 60 minutes, or until a toothpick inserted in the center comes out clean.

Gingered Mushrooms, Bok Choy, and Carrots with Soba Noodles

This is delicious over brown rice, Japanese black rice, or udon noodles. Mirin, a sweetened Japanese rice wine, adds wonderful flavor.

Serves 4

¼ cup mirin
1 tablespoon brown rice vinegar
2 teaspoons low-sodium tamari
2 tablespoons cornstarch
16 ounces mushrooms, sliced
2 carrots, sliced
2 tablespoons fresh ginger, minced
3 cloves garlic, chopped
1 large bunch bok choy, chopped into 2- to 3-inch pieces, or 6 baby bok
    choy
1½ cups vegetable broth
16 ounces soba noodles, cooked
2 tablespoons black sesame seeds

Combine the mirin, brown rice vinegar, tamari, and cornstarch in a small bowl. Stir well and set aside. Stir-fry the mushrooms on medium heat in a skillet or wok for 3 to 4 minutes. Add the carrots, ginger, garlic, and bok choy, and stir-fry for 1 minute. Add the vegetable broth and the mirin mixture, and continue cooking until the bok choy softens and the mixture thickens. Serve over soba noodles and garnish with sesame seeds.

Shepherd's Pie

When I was a kid in Cleveland, a wonderful Yugoslavian neighbor named Mina used to make our family a shepherd's pie several times a year. That pie would hit the top of our lazy Susan dinner table and we six Esselstyns would devour it before the table stopped spinning.

This is almost as good as the original. Savory lentils, green vegetables, and mashed potatoes make it a hearty, satisfying meal.

Serves 4 to 6

3 Yukon Gold potatoes, cut into quarters
½ cup unsweetened plant-based milk
2 tablespoons fresh rosemary, chopped
Cracked pepper to taste
2 cups fresh or frozen green beans
2 onions, diced
½ cup sliced mushrooms
2 cloves garlic, minced
2 cups cooked brown lentils
½ teaspoon ground black pepper
1 tablespoon Bragg Liquid Aminos
6-ounce can tomato paste
1 tablespoon vegetarian Worcestershire sauce

Preheat the oven to 400°F. Steam the potatoes for 15 minutes, until soft. Drain and mash them in a bowl with the plant-based milk, 1 tablespoon of the rosemary, and cracked pepper. Set aside.

Steam the green beans for 7 minutes, or until bright green and still firm. Set aside.

Sauté the onions on medium heat in a large skillet with a few drops of water for 5 minutes, until translucent. Add the mushrooms, garlic, and remaining 1 tablespoon rosemary to the onions. Cook for 5 minutes, until the mushrooms begin to release their juices. Add the lentils, black pepper, and Bragg's. Stir in the tomato paste and Worcestershire sauce, adding a small amount of water as necessary to combine ingredients.

Place the lentil mixture in a skillet or casserole dish. Spread the green beans atop the mixture. Spread the mashed potatoes over the top.

Cover with aluminum foil and bake for 30 minutes. Remove the foil and bake another 5 minutes, or until the potatoes begin to brown lightly.

Variation:
Use frozen peas in place of green beans.

Mac-N-Cash

One of my favorite meals growing up was a plate of frozen Stouffer's macaroni and cheese, which I'd make myself whenever my parents went out to dinner. After cooking it in the oven for 30 minutes, I'd excitedly pull a stool up to our horseshoe-shaped kitchen island and dig in while watching my favorite television program, *The Wild Wild West.* Pure decadence.

I recommend making this for guests and keeping the television off.

Serves 2 to 3

1 onion, chopped
1¼ cup cashews, raw
3 tablespoons lemon juice
1²/₃ cups water
½ teaspoon sea salt
4-ounce jar roasted red peppers, drained
¹/₃ cup nutritional yeast
2 cloves garlic
1 teaspoon onion powder
¼ teaspoon cayenne pepper
16 ounces whole grain elbow pasta, cooked

Preheat the oven to 425°F. Sauté the onion with a few drops of water on medium heat in a skillet for 5 minutes, until translucent. In a food processor, combine the onion, cashews, lemon juice, water, and salt. Gradually blend in the roasted red peppers, nutritional yeast, garlic, onion powder, and cayenne. Thoroughly toss the sauce with the pasta. Bake in a casserole dish in the oven for 20 minutes, until golden brown on top.

E2 Stir-Fries

Stir-fries are fast, easy, simple, and delicious. Loaded with all kinds of fresh vegetables, and served on top of a grain or noodle, they're an Engine 2 MVP. If you want to feel like you're eating a restaurant-quality stir-fry, add a mirin stir-fry sauce (see Stir-Frying, page 136) and bask in each bite. Stir-fries cook quickly over high heat while retaining each vegetable's individual flavor and crispness.

Prep your ingredients before you begin to cook. Place ingredients in separate bowls in the order you will add them to the wok or skillet.

If you like your stir-fries spicy, add a diced jalapeño as the last ingredient.

Vegetable Stir-Fry with Brown Rice

This is an E2 basic because it goes wonderfully over good old-fashioned brown rice—and its taste rules the roost.

Serves 2 to 3

1 pound seitan (Upton brand is good), sliced into strips
½ onion, sliced into half rounds
8 ounces mushrooms, sliced
1 bell pepper, seeded and sliced thin
2 carrots, sliced
2 celery stalks, sliced
8-ounce can sliced water chestnuts, drained
1 clove garlic, minced or pressed
2 tablespoons low-sodium tamari and 1 tablespoon brown sugar, combined
3 cups cooked brown rice (see E2 Brown Rice, page 175)
1 bunch basil for garnish, rinsed and sliced

Heat a large skillet or wok for 3 minutes. Add the seitan, onion, mushrooms, pepper, carrots, celery, water chestnuts, garlic, and the tamari brown sugar combination, stirring for 1 minute after each addition. Serve warm over rice. Garnish with basil.

Tempeh-Mushroom Stir-Fry and Soba Noodles

Tempeh is an unprocessed, whole grain product made from fermented soybeans—unlike tofu and other soybean products, which are usually processed. If you're like me, you'll love its unique taste and texture. It's also very versatile and can be cut, chopped, and crumbled into many dishes. I don't just like it now, I love it!

Serves 2 to 3

16 ounces mugwort soba noodles
8-ounce package tempeh, sliced into thin strips
3 tablespoons low-sodium tamari
Juice of ½ lemon
1 tablespoon whole wheat flour
1 tablespoon molasses
8 shiitake mushrooms, sliced—reconstituted or fresh
8 ounces white mushrooms, sliced
1 clove garlic, minced
2 tablespoons fresh ginger, minced
1 red bell pepper, seeded and sliced thin
1 cup chopped cilantro

Cook the soba noodles per the directions on the package, drain, and set aside. Thoroughly brown the tempeh strips on medium heat in a skillet or wok with 1 tablespoon tamari. Set aside. Mix the remaining 2 tablespoons tamari, lemon juice, flour, and molasses together in a bowl until the flour is dissolved. Set aside. Heat a large skillet or wok until hot Add the remaining ingredients except for the cilantro in the order listed, stirring for 1 minute after each addition. Remove from heat and add the tamari sauce. Serve stir-fry warm over soba noodles and top with tempeh strips. Garnish with cilantro.

Red Vegetable Curry and Brown Rice

There is something about a good curry dish that always keeps me coming back for more. A note of caution: The first time we made this dish at the firehouse, instead of using 1½ tablespoons of the red curry paste, our new driver, Steve Martinez, talked us into using 3. Each of us reacted differently—Steve was in heaven, Scottie was miserable, Matt got the giggles, Derick was cool as a cucumber, and I started sweating profusely.

This dish is spicy! If you prefer something milder, use 1 teaspoon of curry paste.

Serves 2 to 3

Broiled Tofu Cubes
1 pound extra-firm tofu
Bragg Liquid Aminos spray

Curry
2 tablespoons low-sodium tamari
1 tablespoon molasses
1½ tablespoons red curry paste
24 to 32 ounces low-sodium vegetable stock (use 24 if you like your curry thicker, 32 if you like it thinner)
1 onion, sliced into half rounds
3 carrots, sliced into angled rounds
2 cups snow peas
1 cup unsweetened plant-based milk
Juice of 1 lime
3 cups cooked brown rice (see E2 Brown Rice, page 175)
5 green onions, sliced into thin rounds
1 cup cilantro, chopped

For Broiled Tofu Cubes:
Preheat oven to broil. Drain the tofu and cut into 1-inch cubes. Spray the cubes with Bragg's. Broil the cubes on a parchment-lined baking sheet for 20 minutes, flipping them with a spatula once, until browned on both sides.

For Curry:

    Combine the tamari and molasses in a small bowl. Preheat a large skillet or wok with a little water until the water steams Stir-fry the curry paste in ¼ cup of stock, stirring continuously until combined. Add the sliced onion and stir to coat. Add the carrots and snow peas and cook for 1 minute. Add the remaining vegetable stock and the broiled tofu. Stir the tamari mixture into the skillet. Add the plant-based milk and lime juice. Serve curry warm over brown rice. Garnish with sliced green onions and cilantro.

Pad Thai

Two decades ago there was a great vegetarian Thai restaurant in the heart of downtown Austin called Thai Soon. The owner once told me the best way to tell the quality of a Thai restaurant is to sample the pad Thai. If the pad Thai is good, the rest of the dishes probably will be, too.

Serves 3 to 4

3 tablespoons water or low-sodium vegetable stock
1 clove garlic, minced
3 green onions, cut into 1-inch lengths
12 ounces flat rice noodles, soaked in warm water for 20 minutes, then drained
1 recipe Broiled Tofu Cubes (see page 210)
2 cups broccoli florets
1 cup bean sprouts
2 teaspoons dark brown sugar
½ teaspoon chili powder
¼ cup low-sodium tamari
2 tablespoons lemon juice
4 tablespoons home-toasted peanuts, chopped (see Toasting Nuts and
    Seeds, page 139)
8 sprigs cilantro

    Heat the water or vegetable stock in a wok or large skillet until it starts to bubble. Cook the garlic for 1 minute, until the garlic begins to brown lightly. Add the green onions, noodles, tofu, broccoli, and bean sprouts one at a time, stirring for 45 seconds after each addition. Add the sugar, chili powder, tamari, and lemon juice. Stir to combine and remove from heat. Garnish with peanuts and cilantro.

E2 Big Salads

The great thing about these big salads is they are big on taste and substance and have very little air. Every bite is hearty, substantial, and bustling with flavor. Best of all, you don't have to drown them with dressing—in fact, the lighter your dressing touch, the better!

Rice Salad

This satisfying salad is the perfect marriage of grains, beans, vegetables, and fruit. Serve on top of a bed of field greens with a side of healthy corn chips.

Serves 2 to 3

3 cups cooked brown rice (see E2 Brown Rice, page 175)
16-ounce can pinto beans, rinsed and drained
15-ounce can corn, rinsed and drained
2 bell peppers, seeded and chopped
4 green onions, chopped
¼ cup raisins
1 cup cilantro, chopped
¼ cup fruit or balsamic vinegar
Cracked pepper to taste
¼ cup home-toasted walnuts (see Toasting Nuts and Seeds, page 139)

Toss all the ingredients except the pepper and nuts together in a large bowl. Season with the pepper. Sprinkle the walnuts over the salad before serving.

Variations:
Spice it up with a diced jalapeño. Serve with avocado slices and salsa.

Spinach Salad with Healthy Homemade Croutons

Spinach is one of the most nutritionally dense foods you can eat. Low in calories and high in quality, spinach is an E2 all-star. Popeye was definitely in the know! No wonder he always got Olive Oyl. Poor Brutus—he ate too much meat.

Serves 2

2 cups whole grain bread cut into 1-inch squares
Bragg Liquid Aminos spray
1 tablespoon dried parsley
1 teaspoon garlic powder
1 teaspoon onion powder
1 teaspoon paprika
Cracked pepper to taste
1 red onion, sliced into half rounds
½ cup home-toasted walnuts (see Toasting Nuts and Seeds, page 139)
2 tablespoons maple syrup
1 tablespoon balsamic vinegar
1 pound bag fresh spinach, thoroughly rinsed
15-ounce can chickpeas, rinsed and drained
1 cucumber, sliced into thin rounds
Sesame Seed Dressing (see page 233)

For Croutons:

Preheat the oven to broil. Spray the bread cubes lightly with Bragg's and toss with the parsley, garlic and onion powders, paprika, and cracked pepper. Broil seasoned bread cubes on a baking sheet, flipping them with a spatula once, after 1 to 2 minutes, until browned on both sides. Toasting croutons takes only a few minutes, depending upon how dry the bread is—take care not to burn them!

For Caramelized Onion and Walnuts:

Cook the onion on high heat in a skillet with a few drops of water for 5 to 8 minutes, until the slices begin to brown. Add the walnuts and cook for another 3 minutes, stirring frequently, until they begin to crisp. Add the maple syrup and vinegar and stir frequently for 1 minute, or until the liquid bubbles and coats the contents.

For Assembling the Salad:

Toss the spinach with the chickpeas, cucumber, and onions and walnuts. Dress the salad with Sesame Seed Dressing and top with croutons.

Variations:

Personalize the croutons by using dried or fresh herbs of your choice in place of the parsley: tarragon, thyme, oregano, and rosemary are good alternatives.

Add sliced tomatoes, carrots, and bell pepper strips.

Use any no-fat salad dressing of your choice.

Save stale bread to make batches of croutons, and make extras to freeze. They are delicious with any salad or soup.

The Great Wooden Bowl Salad

One of Jill's and my best wedding presents was a big wooden salad bowl brimming with character, a gift from my parents. The first Engine 2 Pilot Study potluck dinner was held in February 2007, and because I wanted to honor the bowl by filling it with something wonderfully special, I packed it from top to bottom with this beast of a salad that was as big a hit as the bowl itself.

Serves 3 to 4

¼ cup nutritional yeast
½ teaspoon garlic powder
1 pound extra-firm tofu, drained and cut into mini squares ½ x ½ inch
½ cup walnuts
Bragg Liquid Aminos spray
1 head romaine lettuce, torn into chunks
8 ounces cherry or grape tomatoes
4 carrots, sliced into rounds
4 stalks celery, sliced
1 cup arugula
½ cup cilantro, chopped
15-ounce can black beans, drained and rinsed
2 grapefruits, peeled into sections
Cracked pepper to taste
E2 salad dressing of choice (see pages 232–234)

For Tofu:

Mix the nutritional yeast and garlic powder on a plate. Press the tofu pieces into the mixture to coat. Sauté the tofu in a skillet on high heat for 3 minutes on each side, or until nicely browned. Remove to a bowl. Wipe the skillet with a cloth to use for the walnuts.

For Walnuts:

Spray the walnuts with Bragg's. Cook in a medium-high heat skillet, stirring constantly for 3 minutes, or until browned.

For Assembling Salad:

Place the romaine lettuce pieces into a large bowl. Top with the cooked tofu and remaining ingredients, using the walnuts as the final garnish. Toss thoroughly with the E2 salad dressing of your choice.

Rip's Roasted Salad

The largest salad in the world was tossed in Spain in 2007 with the help of twenty cooks working for more than three hours. Guinness World Records was officially on hand to weigh in the heavyweight champion at a staggering 14,740 pounds.

This big salad takes less time to prepare and there won't be nearly as many leftovers.

Serves 3 to 4

12 Brussels sprouts, cut in half
1 head cauliflower, cut into florets
8 ounces new potatoes, cut in half
1 onion, sliced into rounds
1 head romaine lettuce, torn into chunks
15-ounce can corn, rinsed and drained
1 red bell pepper, seeded and sliced
11-ounce can mandarin oranges, drained
E2 salad dressing of choice (see pages 232–234)

For Roasting Vegetables:

Preheat the oven to 475°F. Place the Brussels sprouts, cauliflower florets, potato halves, and onion slices cut-side down on one or more large parchment-lined baking sheets. Broil the vegetables for 15 minutes or longer, until browning on the tops. Check frequently for burning. Allow the vegetables to cool to room temperature.

For Assembling Salad:

Put the romaine lettuce pieces in a large bowl. Cover with the roasted vegetables. Top with the corn, bell pepper, and mandarin oranges. Toss thoroughly with the E2 salad dressing of your choice.

E2 Soups

Soup can be thin and light or thick and hearty. Engine 2 soups are usually the latter. They often are hearty enough to serve as an entire meal, even for people who think of them as an appetizer. Soup is just the best.

I recommend adding greens to your soup about three minutes before you ladle yourself a bowl to turn it into a power soup. When the soup is good, all is good!

Split Pea Soup

Split peas are 22 percent protein and a great source of soluble fiber. Serve this hearty soup alone, or atop a bed of chopped spinach, arugula, and cooked brown rice, with healthy crackers or whole grain toast.

Serves 3 to 4

1 onion, chopped
2 bay leaves
2 cloves garlic, minced or pressed
16 ounces dried split peas, rinsed and drained
4 cups low-sodium vegetable stock
3 cups water
6 Yukon Gold potatoes, diced
2 tablespoons Bragg Liquid Aminos
4 stalks celery with leaves, chopped
4 carrots, chopped
1 cup parsley, chopped
1 teaspoon ground thyme, or 4 sprigs fresh
1 tablespoon white vinegar
Cracked black or ground white pepper to taste

Sauté the onion and bay leaves on high heat in a soup pot with a few drops of water for 5 minutes, until the onion browns. Add the garlic and split peas, stirring for 3 minutes, until warm. Add the vegetable stock, water, diced potatoes, and Bragg's, and bring to a boil. Cover and cook over low heat, stirring occasionally, for 30 minutes. Add warm water as necessary to achieve desired consistency. Add the celery, carrots, parsley, thyme, and vinegar, and cook for 5 to 10 minutes. Continue to cook until the peas achieve the desired consistency. Season with pepper.

Mexican Lime Soup

This soup is fun to offer guests. Serve it in large bowls, and crumble healthy chips on top of the soup before enjoying.

Serves 4 to 6

1 large onion, chopped
8 ounces mushrooms, cut into quarters
2 bay leaves
2 cloves garlic, minced or pressed
3 roasted poblano chili peppers (see Roasting Peppers and Fresh Chilies,
    page 139), cut into strips
2 to 3 (32-ounce) cartons low-sodium vegetable stock
2 ears of corn, husks removed, cut into 2-inch rounds
4 medium red potatoes, cut into 1-inch cubes
1 bunch cilantro, chopped
3 limes
4 tomatoes, chopped
2 avocados, peeled and sliced
Corn chips (see E2-Approved Foods to Keep in Your Pantry, page 127)

For Soup:

Sauté the onion, garlic, mushrooms, and bay leaves on medium heat in a large soup pot with a few drops of water for 5 minutes, until the onion browns. Add the roasted chili peppers and 1 cup of stock. Stir intermittently for 5 minutes, until the peppers begin to soften. Add the corn, potatoes, and the remaining stock until all the vegetables are submerged in liquid by 1 inch. Cook on high heat until it comes to a boil and then reduce heat to medium-low and cover for 15 to 20 minutes, until the potatoes are tender. Remove from heat and let sit covered for 5 minutes.

For Serving:

Stir the cilantro, zest of 1 lime, and the juice of 3 limes into the soup immediately before serving. Place a handful each of tomatoes, avocados, and corn chips into large soup bowls. Pour the hot soup directly over the vegetables and chips and serve.

Variations:

Use 8 ounces of canned green chilies in place of fresh poblanos.

Use a 1-pound bag of frozen corn in place of fresh corn (preferably roasted).

Kole's Creamy Cauliflower Soup

My son, Kole, loves this wonderful soup. It was served at our friends Mark and Monica Cravotta's Christmas Day potluck dinner, and Kole went to town on it. My wife, Jill, then perfected this tasty and surprisingly rich soup to make it a cinch to prepare. This recipe is great as is—or, as I often prefer, doubled for even more terrific soup!

Serves 6

2 large onions, chopped
½ teaspoon sea salt
2½ cups water
8 yukon gold potatoes, chopped
½ cup chopped celery
2 large carrots, diced
1 head cauliflower, cut into bite-size florets
2 cups vegetable broth (or enough to submerge vegetables by ½ inch)
2 tablespoons no-oil-added cashew or peanut butter
2 tablespoons low-sodium tamari
1 cup nutritional yeast
Sea salt and cracked pepper to taste

Heat the onion, salt, and ½ cup water in a large soup pot on high heat for 5 minutes, then simmer on low for approximately 20 minutes, or until the onions cook down to a nice mush. Check to make sure the water is sufficient, and adding ¼ cup of water as needed so the onions don't burn on the bottom of the pot.

Add the potatoes, celery, carrots, and cauliflower along with 2 cups of water and the vegetable broth. Simmer until all the vegetables are soft—about 20 minutes.

Add the cashew butter and tamari. Mash with a potato masher (or blend with an immersion blender) until the soup is mostly smooth, with some nice chunks. Stir in 1 cup of nutritional yeast. Season with cracked pepper and sea salt.

Variations:

Add one bunch of freshly chopped kale, mustard greens, or collard greens 5 to 8 minutes before serving for a nutritional power punch!

Three-Bean Chili

Matt and Steve were on vacation and Scottie wasn't around. Therefore, it was just Derick and me at the station for the C shift on a warm April day, along with two travelers (travelers are firefighters who come from other stations to fill in during absences).

I asked them if they'd like to join us for our plant-bold dinner wagon. "Absolutely!" they both said.

So I cooked up my three-bean chili. The travelers enjoyed the meal so much they thought they might just eat plant-based all the time. But three hours later, while sitting on the porch outside the station, they were hit by some unexpected flatulence. Derick and I, whose systems are acclimated to this healthy, cleansing food, were fine.

Keep in mind, some people will have a lag time of a few weeks before their gastrointestinal tract settles into happiness. However, as your body gets used to the enormous amount of roughage in the E2 Diet, you will soon be as silent as the night, as regular as Big Ben, and feel zero stomach distress.

Serve this chili on top of a bed of fresh greens with warm whole grain tortillas or healthy chips. For an even heartier meal, serve over brown rice and greens.

Serves 6 to 8

1 large onion, chopped
2 cloves garlic, minced or pressed

2 bay leaves
2 green bell peppers, seeded and chopped
2 stalks celery, chopped
2 carrots, chopped
1 cup chopped mushrooms
1 jalapeño pepper, chopped (remove the ribs and seeds to reduce heat)
15-ounce can kidney beans, rinsed and drained
15-ounce can black beans, rinsed and drained
15-ounce can chickpeas, rinsed and drained
3 cups water
2 28-ounce cans plum tomatoes, with juice, chopped
6-ounce can tomato paste
1 pound firm tofu, drained and crumbled
15-ounce can corn, rinsed and drained
1 apple, chopped
2 tablespoons chili powder
2 teaspoons coriander
2 tablespoons Dijon mustard
1 tablespoon molasses
½ cup chopped parsley or cilantro
Sea salt and cracked pepper to taste

Sauté onion on medium-high heat in a large soup pot with a few drops of water for 5 minutes. Add garlic, bay leaves, bell peppers, celery, carrots, mushrooms, and jalapeño, then cook on medium for 5 more minutes. Add the beans, water, tomatoes, tomato paste, tofu, corn, apple, spices, mustard, molasses, and parsley. Cover and simmer on low heat for 15 to 20 minutes. Season with salt and pepper.

Variations:
Garnish with sliced avocado, chopped raw onion, minced jalapeños, Southwest Salsa (see page 240), or E2 Sour Cream (see page 239).
Add cooked lentils to the pot with the beans and tomatoes.

Savory Lentils and Greens

With all the greens in this, it is hard to find a healthier soup. And it's quick, because the lentils can be served al dente. If you prefer them soupy-thick, cook them a little longer, stirring frequently. At Engine 2, we like the small green French lentils, but don't forget to give the yellow, brown, and orange lentils a shot as well.

Serve with warm whole grain bread or brown rice and greens.

Serves a firehouse of 10

2 medium onions, chopped
2 stalks celery, chopped
4 cloves garlic, chopped
3 carrots, chopped
4 tomatoes, chopped
2½ cups uncooked lentils
5 cups vegetable broth
5 cups water
Cracked pepper to taste
2 large heads of leafy greens, chopped into bite-size pieces. Use kale, collards, spinach, Swiss chard, or a combination of as many as you wish.

In a large soup pot, add onion, celery, garlic, and carrots and cook over low heat for 10 minutes, stirring frequently. Add the tomatoes and cook for 5 more minutes. Add the lentils, broth, water, and pepper, turn the heat up to high, and bring to a boil uncovered. Cover, turn the heat down to low, and simmer for 45 minutes. Add the greens and simmer for another 10 minutes or, for especially green and fresh-looking greens, boil or steam the greens first, then add them to the soup pot just before serving.

E2 Tex-Mex Favorites

Tex-Mex cuisine, which blends Texan and Mexican food, has become quite popular throughout the country, but in Austin, it's probably the most common cuisine around: tortillas, wraps, burritos, enchiladas, tacos, salsas, and sauces.

Traditionally, all these favorites are stuffed with different meats and cheeses. This is where E2 breaks from Tex-Mex tradition—yet we have discovered that Tex-Mex, with E2 modifications, can be as healthy as it is delicious.

E2 Basics Tacos

Tacos are a snap to prepare—but make sure you are using corn rather than flour tortillas. Corn tortillas contain no oil and are fat-free. This allows you to eat several more while taking in fewer calories: more of the good stuff, less of the bad.

Be inventive. Find your favorite combinations. Go taco crazy.

Serves 2

6 corn tortillas
15-ounce can black beans, rinsed and drained
½ cup water
1 teaspoon chili powder
1 avocado, sliced, or Guacamole (see page 238)
1 cup shredded romaine lettuce
Salsa (see page 240)

Warm the tortillas (see Warming Tortillas and Wraps, page 139). Heat the beans, water, and chili powder in a saucepan at medium heat for 5 minutes. Mash the beans with a potato masher. Spoon the beans and avocado onto warm tortillas. Sprinkle with lettuce, season with salsa, and roll into burritos.

Variations for Fillings:
Tex-Mex leftovers
Sweet potato, cilantro, and pan-fried mushrooms
Pinto beans and Southwest Salsa (see page 240)
Broiled Tofu Cubes (see page 210) with shredded romaine lettuce and salsa

Picadillo Pick Ax Burrito

Picadillo is a traditional beef taco filling that makes a terrific complement to potatoes, beans, and/or rice. Think of it as a cute little burrito.

We've simplified the recipe to create a healthy E2 version.

Serves 4

1 onion, diced
15-ounce can no-salt-added black beans
¼ cup water
1 teaspoon Bragg Liquid Aminos
2 tablespoons chili powder
1 tablespoon ground cumin
4 whole grain wraps or 8 corn tortillas
15-ounce can corn, rinsed and drained
2 tomatoes, diced
3 cups shredded romaine lettuce
Salsa (see page 240)

In a skillet with a few drops of water on high heat, sauté the onion for 3 minutes or until translucent. Add the beans, water, Bragg's, and spices. Cook on medium-high heat for 10 minutes, or until the water is absorbed and the mixture is browning. Warm the wraps or tortillas. Fill the wraps with the black bean mixture, corn, tomatoes, a generous handful of lettuce, and salsa, and roll into burritos.

Variations:

Leftover potatoes can be quickly sautéed in a skillet with green onions or bell peppers, and the mixture added to a burrito. Serve with Guacamole (see page 238), minced jalapeño, chopped raw onion or tomatoes, salsa, rice, or beans.

Rip's Tip

To make "fried" taco shells, hang corn tortillas over one or two of the metal bars in your oven and bake at 350°F for 4 minutes or until crispy. Check frequently.

Chalupas

Traditionally, chalupas are corn tortillas fried in oil until crispy and topped with beans, meat, and cheese. Our healthy E2 chalupas are easy to prepare and even more delicious. You can definitely eat these with your fingers!

Serves 2

6 corn tortillas
16-ounce can fat-free vegetarian refried beans
12 cherry tomatoes, cut in half
1 jalapeño, diced (remove the ribs and seeds to reduce heat)
1 avocado, peeled and sliced
2 cups shredded romaine lettuce
½ bunch cilantro, chopped
Salsa (see page 240)

Preheat the oven to broil. Place the tortillas on a parchment-lined baking sheet and broil for 2 minutes. Turn the tortillas and broil for 1 minute, or until crispy. Spread the tortillas thickly with beans. Place 4 tomato halves on each chalupa. Sprinkle jalapeño onto the chalupas. Return to the oven and broil for 5 to 7 minutes, or until the tomatoes begin to droop. Divide the avocado slices among the chalupas and top with the lettuce, salsa, and cilantro.

Variations:
Drizzle chalupas with E2 Sour Cream (see page 239) before serving.

Nachos

Leftover nachos are like leftover pizza—delicious cold!

Serves 4

8 to 10 corn tortillas, cut in 1-inch squares and toasted, or 1 bag fat-free
 baked corn chips
2 (15-ounce) cans black beans, rinsed and drained
2 large tomatoes, diced
1 bell pepper, seeded and diced
4 green onions, sliced into rounds
Salsa (see page 240)
Guacamole (see page 238)
2 cups shredded romaine lettuce

Preheat the oven to broil. Spread the tortilla squares or chips across a parchment-lined baking sheet. Spoon the beans over the chips. Add the tomatoes, bell pepper, and green onions. Bake until the chips are slightly browned on the edges, 7 to 10 minutes. Using a spatula, push the nachos onto a large serving plate. Top with salsa, guacamole, and romaine lettuce.

Variations:
Drizzle E2 Sour Cream (see page 239) over the cooked nachos.
Use warm refried beans in place of black beans.
Add sliced jalapeños to the mound of nachos before cooking.

Rip's Sweet Potato Bowl

I love this simple and fast dinner bowl. Filled with all kinds of nutritious and delicious ingredients, it has a great variety of tastes and colors, and is truly satisfying.

I always keep a few cooked sweet potatoes in the fridge so I can pop them in the microwave for 3 to 4 minutes while chopping up the other ingredients. Dinner is done in less than 6 minutes!

Serves 2

1 large cooked sweet potato, skin removed, cut into cubes
1 mango, peeled, seeded, and cut into cubes
1 red bell pepper, seeded and chopped
15-ounce can black beans, rinsed and drained
1 avocado, peeled, seeded, and chopped
½ bunch cilantro, chopped
Juice of 1 lime
Balsamic vinegar to taste

Warm the sweet potatoes in a microwave if using chilled leftovers. Place a generous portion of sweet potatoes into a large serving bowl. Top with mango, bell pepper, beans, avocado, and cilantro. Drizzle with lime juice and vinegar, stir gently, and serve.

EMS Portobello Mushroom Fajitas with Rice and Guacamole

One evening, after wrapping up a car accident scene with EMS, the paramedics asked when we were going to invite them over for an Engine 2 dinner. We told them we had plenty of leftovers, and it was now or never. They happily raced the ambulance over to the station and polished off the rest of our fajitas, which we had actually been saving for lunch. But it never hurts to be friends with the local paramedics.

This is one of E2's signature dinners—and signature leftover dishes.

Serves 4

4 Portobello mushrooms, sliced into thick strips
1 large onion, sliced
2 bell peppers, seeded and sliced into thin strips
1 jalapeño pepper, diced (remove the ribs and seeds to reduce heat)
12 corn or whole grain tortillas
Guacamole (see page 238)
Salsa (see page 240)
3 cups cooked brown rice (see E2 Brown Rice, page 175)
15-ounce can no-salt-added black beans

Cook the mushrooms in a large skillet with a little water on high heat for 3 minutes, or until the mushrooms begin to brown slightly. Add the onion to the skillet and cook for 5 minutes. Add the bell peppers and jalapeño and cook for 3 minutes. Warm the tortillas (see Warming Tortillas and Wraps, page 139). To serve, spoon the vegetables into the corn tortillas and top with guacamole and salsa. Serve with a side of rice and beans.

Variation:
Serve with pinto beans and E2 Sour Cream (see page 239).

Jane's Jammin' Burritos

These are another of my sister Jane's many plant-happy creations. Her nickname is Jungle Jane because she wears crazy outfits and has a crazy thick mane of blond hair. Her burritos are a testament to her jungle of love for plant-bursting foods. These stick to your ribs like nobody's business.

Serves 6

1 large onion, chopped
2 cloves garlic, minced
2 zucchini, chopped
2 yellow squash, chopped
1 red bell pepper, seeded and chopped
3 cups shredded napa cabbage
2 15-ounce cans black beans, rinsed and drained
2 15-ounce cans fat-free vegetarian refried beans
1 cup cooked brown rice (see E2 Brown Rice, page 175)
2 teaspoons ground cumin
⅛ teaspoon cayenne pepper
6 large Ezekiel 4:9 sprouted-grain tortillas
Salsa (see page 240)
Guacamole (see page 238)

Preheat the oven to 350°F. Sauté the onion and garlic in a large skillet with a few drops of water on high heat for 3 minutes. Turn the heat down to medium and add the zucchini, yellow squash, bell pepper, and cabbage to the skillet. Cook 4 to 5 minutes, stirring occasionally until the vegetables are al dente (soft but firm) and the cabbage is wilting. Add the black beans, refried beans, and rice to the skillet. Reduce the heat to low and stir the ingredients together until the mixture is thick and mortar-like. Season with the cumin and cayenne.

Slap a large spoonful of veggie mortar onto the center of a tortilla and spread it from top to bottom along the center line. Fold the sides over using a bit of the veggie mortar as adhesive for the top flap. Rest the burritos next to each other and place them seam-side down on a parchment-lined baking sheet. Bake for 20 minutes or until the wraps are crisp. Serve with salsa and guacamole on top.

Matt Moore's Enchiladas

One day, Engine 2 firefighter Matt Moore started talking about how he'd just had an intense dream about a raging house fire. Since Matt seldom says such things, it made us all think we were about to face a real burner.

We went on several calls that day, but none of them were fires. Then, at 6:30 that evening, as Matt was putting his enchiladas into the oven, the tone sounded for a church fire on the east side.

It turned out to be a tough call. After being on air and doing salvage and overhaul work for nearly thirty minutes in 100-degree heat, all of us were sent to rehab. Scottie didn't look good—he was red in the face and his eyes were bloodshot. EMS examined him and decided he was suffering from dehydration with a bit of heat exhaustion—nothing that a liter of fluid couldn't remedy.

We had to endure snide comments from various firefighters about how we needed to feed him more meat: "Give that boy a steak," or "Put some chicken broth in that IV." At the debriefing, even the incident commander said, "Well, nobody got hurt except Scottie Walters, and all he needs is a little more protein."

When we made it back to the station, after agreeing that sarcasm and ignorance get a lot of people pretty far in this world, we finally got around to eating. But before any of us took a bite, we all offered a toast to Matt and his tasty meat-free enchiladas, as well as his dreams.

Incidentally, this was originally my recipe, which Matt stole, perfected, and made into his signature dish. He's not a fan of onions: When it's his turn to cook, he avoids them like the plague. When I cook? Everything starts with an onion.

Serve enchiladas with a starter salad.

Serves 6

2 cups sliced mushrooms, sliced
4 cups thawed and drained frozen spinach,
30-ounce package fat-free, frozen hash brown potatoes
2 tablespoons chili powder
2 teaspoons ground cumin
8-ounce can diced green chilies
18 corn tortillas
3 16-ounce jars enchilada sauce
12 sprigs cilantro

Preheat the oven to 425°F. Sauté the mushrooms and spinach on medium heat in a large skillet with a little water for 5 minutes, or until the mushrooms are soft. Drain the liquid, and remove the mushrooms and spinach to a large bowl. Cook the potatoes on high heat in a skillet for 10 minutes until lightly browned on both sides. Sprinkle with chili powder and cumin. Add the potatoes and green chilies to the bowl with the mushrooms and spinach and gently combine. Line the bottom of a 9-by-13-inch casserole dish with parchment and lay 6 tortillas on the bottom. Place half of the vegetable mixture over the tortillas and cover with one jar of sauce. Repeat the process: tortillas, vegetables, sauce. Top with the remaining six tortillas and jar of sauce. Bake uncovered for 30 minutes. Allow to sit for 15 minutes before serving. Garnish with the cilantro sprigs.

E2 POP QUIZ

Q: If you eat 100 calories from complex carbohydrates and 100 calories from fat, how many of those calories get burned up digesting, absorbing, and storing the food you've just eaten?

A: If you've eaten 100 calories from carbohydrates, 25 of the 100 calories are burned up in the storage process. If you've eaten 100 calories from fat, only 2 get burned up in the storage process.

E2 DRESSINGS, SPREADS, AND MARINADES

Dressings make or break a salad. I have yet to find a really good store-bought salad dressing that can measure up to the tough E2 standards of health and taste. So instead try our homemade recipes—they are delicious and each yields about ½ cup.

E2 Basics Dressing

This is one of my favorite salad dressings. My wonderful friend Bridget, who introduced me to the many wonders of vegetarian cooking, whipped it up for me one night in 1996, and my salads have been grateful ever since.

2 tablespoons nutritional yeast
2 tablespoons balsamic vinegar
1 tablespoon low-sodium tamari
1 tablespoon mustard
Juice of 1 orange, lime, or lemon
1 tablespoon maple syrup
1 teaspoon vegetarian Worcestershire sauce
1 tablespoon wheat germ
Water to desired consistency

Whisk the ingredients together in a bowl.

Dijon Dressing

Our healthy version of a classic Dijon vinaigrette.

½ cup seasoned rice vinegar
1 to 2 teaspoons Dijon mustard
1 clove garlic, minced or pressed

Whisk the ingredients together in a bowl.

Peanut Dressing

One of Austin's veteran firefighters is nicknamed Peanut because when he attended the fire academy at the age of nineteen, he was only five feet, six inches tall and he weighed 150 pounds. An instructor gave him the name and it stuck. Over the next several years the man grew six inches and he now weighs close to 230 pounds. Everyone still calls him Peanut—even his wife.

Here's a peanut dressing that's also hefty in terms of taste, kick—and fat. Remember, nuts are nutritional powerhouses, but they're not low-fat!

3 tablespoons chunky no-oil-added peanut butter
3 tablespoons maple syrup
2 tablespoons cider vinegar
1 tablespoon water

Whisk the ingredients together in a bowl.

Variations:
Add ½ teaspoon chopped jalapeño or serrano pepper.
Add black pepper or crushed red pepper to taste.
Add 2 tablespoons chopped green onion.

Sesame Seed Dressing

This dressing is surprising in its hearty, satisfying flavor. An old Southern favorite, this is just the ticket for topping fresh spinach.

3 tablespoons home-toasted sesame seeds (see Toasting Nuts and Seeds, page 139)
2 tablespoons maple syrup
2 tablespoons low-sodium tamari
Smidge of water

Whisk the ingredients together in a bowl.

Orange Hummus Dressing

Possibly the most delicious dressing of all.

3 tablespoons Healthy Homemade Hummus (see page 236)
3 tablespoons orange juice
2 tablespoons balsamic vinegar
1 teaspoon mustard
½ teaspoon minced ginger

Whisk the ingredients together in a bowl.

Creamy Green Avocado Dressing

This creamy avocado dressing is as smooth as silk and tantalizingly tasty.

¼ package firm Mori-Nu silken tofu
1 avocado, peeled and seeded
Juice of ½ lime

Blend the ingredients together until smooth, adding a small amount of unsweetened plant-based milk or water to achieve the desired consistency.

Beam Me Up, Scottie, Dressing

Fellow E2 firefighter and pal Scottie Walters invented this dressing with three ingredients we found lying around the station. It has since become a firehouse favorite.

3 tablespoons balsamic vinegar
2 tablespoons mustard
1 tablespoon maple syrup
Smidge of water

Whisk the ingredients together in a bowl.

* * *

Now that you're leaving mayonnaise and other disastrous condiments behind, it's time to find healthy and suitable replacements. Many Engine 2 participants are convinced they would not have been successful if it weren't for these healthy homemade spreads, which are easy to make and can be used for sandwiches and wraps or as dips for chips, crackers, and vegetables. They will keep in the refrigerator for up to one week. Each recipe makes about 2 cups, unless otherwise noted.

Black Bean Spread

Black beans are incredibly versatile. This spread is one of many ways black beans make their presence felt in the E2 diet.

15-ounce can black beans, rinsed and drained
1 clove garlic, coarsely chopped
¼ teaspoon ground cumin
¼ teaspoon sea salt
3 tablespoons unsweetened plant-based milk
Juice of 1 small lime

Blend all the ingredients together until combined.

Variation:

To spice up your black bean spread, add to the above ingredients 1 tablespoon chili powder, 1 seeded and chopped jalapeño, and 1 small red onion, diced and sautéed on medium heat for 5 minutes.

Healthy Homemade Hummus

This is the most basic of the spreads. You can find a variation of this recipe in almost any grocery store, but 95 percent of them are made with either olive oil or tahini (sesame paste), which pushes up the fat content. Your best bet is to take 3 minutes and make a batch on Sunday that will last you for the week.

15-ounce can chickpeas, rinsed and drained
2 cloves garlic, chopped
2 to 3 tablespoons fresh lemon juice
1 teaspoon Bragg Liquid Aminos or low-sodium tamari
3 tablespoons water or vegetable broth

Blend all the ingredients into a thick paste, using additional amounts of water or vegetable broth to achieve the desired consistency.

Variations:
Customize by adding one or more of the following:

2 tablespoons home-toasted sesame seeds (see Toasting Nuts and Seeds, page 139)
1 fresh jalapeño, seeded and chopped
1 roasted red bell pepper (see Roasting Peppers and Fresh Chilies, page 139)
1 cup dark or Kalamata olives
1 bunch fresh mint
1 cup fresh spinach
1 cup cooked eggplant

Kale Butter

This spread was invented by my sister, Jane, who is always looking for creative ways to get greens into her kids' diet. This recipe works so well that before long your kids will be asking you for the kale butter instead of peanut butter.

Use kale butter as a spread for crackers or wraps.

1 bunch kale, rinsed, destemmed, and chopped (see Preparing Leafy Greens, page 140)
½ cup walnuts
Sea salt to taste

Steam the kale for 5 minutes, until tender. Reserve the steaming water. Blend the cooked kale with the walnuts and ½ cup of the green water from steaming. Add salt if desired. Process in a blender until smooth.

Cannellini Dip

Cannellini beans are smooth and satiating, and this dip does the trick with one quick spin in the Cuisinart.

15-ounce can cannellini beans, rinsed and drained
1 clove garlic, coarsely chopped
Juice of 1 lemon
¼ teaspoon dried thyme
¼ teaspoon dried rosemary
¼ teaspoon sea salt
Cracked pepper to taste

Blend all the ingredients until they form a paste.

Variation:
Add 4 coarsely chopped Kalamata olives.

Tofu Vegetable Spread

So hearty and delicious you can use it as you would a tuna or egg salad.

½ pound extra-firm tofu, drained and crumbled
Juice of ½ lemon
1 teaspoon dried mustard
1½ teaspoons white vinegar
¼ teaspoon turmeric
¼ teaspoon paprika
¼ teaspoon sea salt
Cracked pepper to taste

Process all the ingredients until slightly chunky, about 15 seconds.

Variations:

Customize by stirring one or more of the following into the processed spread:

2 thinly sliced green onions
1 sliced rib celery
3 tablespoons pickle relish
¼ cup diced white onion

Guacamole

Man, guacamole is good—but it's not for those trying to lose weight or lower their cholesterol numbers. Avocados, loaded with nutrients, are also loaded with calories and fat. That's why we use a cucumber to add volume and lessen the amount of fat in each serving.

2 avocados, seeded and peeled
1 clove garlic, minced or pressed
1 tomato, chopped
¼ onion, diced
1 cucumber, seeded and diced
Juice of 1 lime
½ cup chopped cilantro

Combine the ingredients with a potato masher or fork. For presentation and to preserve the green color of the avocados, place one avocado seed atop the guacamole.

Variations:

For a simpler version, mash 2 avocados with the juice of 1 lime and 1 clove minced garlic.

Add 1 teaspoon chili powder or chili sauce.

E2 Sour Cream

Often, it's not what people choose as their main course that matters, but what they choose to put on top of it. Fat-laden, artery-clogging sour cream is a perfect example—of the wrong choice. Belly up to the trough with this excellent E2 Sour Cream and make that enchilada or taco much tastier and much, much healthier.

Makes 2½ cups

1 package lite firm silken tofu
⅓ cup unsweetened plant-based milk
3 tablespoons lemon or lime juice
2 tablespoons chopped cilantro or dill
1 tablespoon nutritional yeast

Blend all the ingredients together until smooth. Cover and chill for 1 hour before serving to allow the flavors to blend.

Salsa

When I first arrived in Texas as a kid from Cleveland, Ohio, I had no idea what salsa was. I knew only two condiments: ketchup and mustard. But after living here for thirty-five years, I've come to love a good salsa more than any other sauce.

This one's an Engine 2 specialty. We often whip it up first thing when we come on shift at high noon, and then snack on it throughout the day along with healthy crackers, pita bread, or toasted corn tortillas.

14.5-ounce can tomatoes
1 large jalapeño pepper, diced (remove the ribs and seeds to reduce heat)
2 cloves garlic, coarsely chopped
1 cup cilantro
2 green onions, coarsely chopped
Juice of 1 lime

Blend the ingredients together to achieve the desired consistency.

Variations:

This salsa can be served fresh, or simmered on low heat for 20 minutes and served either at room temperature or chilled. Six small fresh tomatoes can be substituted for the canned tomatoes.

Southwest Salsa

This chunky salsa is a great complement to wraps and tacos, and also wonderful on top of beans and rice.

2 large carrots, grated
1 red bell pepper, seeded and chopped
1 cucumber, cut into quarters, seeded, and diced
4 green onions, chopped
½ cup chopped cilantro
1 clove garlic, minced
1 jalapeño pepper, minced (optional)
4 tablespoons white vinegar
1 tablespoon molasses

Place the carrots, bell pepper, cucumber, green onions, cilantro, garlic, and jalapeño in a bowl. Mix the vinegar and molasses together and toss with vegetables.

Rip's Tip

Southwest Salsa is better on the second day, and keeps well in the refrigerator for up to a week.

MANY TIMES SPICES TAKE YOU only so far. That's when it's nice to have the option of calling in a reinforcement such as a marinade. A marinade is a blend of ingredients that, combined with vegetables, tofu, or meat, acts as a great flavor enhancer. The key is to allow the food to soak in the marinade so it can penetrate deep inside.

The instructions for these marinades are all the same: Mix all the ingredients thoroughly in a sealed container or plastic baggie. Add tofu and shake to coat. Allow to marinate refrigerated for 30 minutes to 4 hours.

Asian Marinade

Juice of 2 lemons
3 tablespoons low-sodium soy sauce
1 tablespoon grated fresh ginger, or 1 teaspoon dried
1 tablespoon molasses (more to taste)
Cracked pepper to taste, or ½ teaspoon seeded, minced jalapeño

Island Marinade

1 8-ounce can crushed pineapple, undrained
¼ cup low-sodium soy sauce
2 tablespoons molasses
Red pepper flakes to taste

Mexican Marinade

Juice of 2 or 3 limes
2 tablespoons Bragg Liquid Aminos
2 tablespoons brown sugar
½ cup chopped cilantro (more to taste)
½ teaspoon seeded, minced jalapeño

Continental Marinade

½ cup white wine
¼ cup country-style Dijon mustard
¼ cup maple syrup
2 tablespoons Bragg Liquid Aminos
½ cup chopped dill or 2 tablespoons chopped thyme
Cracked pepper to taste

Celia Sanchez, 40, Jessica Sanchez, 23
Mother and Daughter

Celia: I came down with ovarian cancer and my doctor recommended I eat a plant-based diet. So I decided to go on Rip's diet—and my daughter decided that she wanted to support me by doing it, too. It wasn't as hard as either of us thought. But both of us had to learn how to cook differently.

Jessica: All in all, I lost thirteen pounds, and even better, before starting the diet, I had kidney stones. They went away!

Celia: I'm also grateful because I used to go to the bathroom three times a week—now I go three times a day. That feels great, too!

SNACKS

Like most people, I love to snack. When I was a triathlete, training four to eight hours and burning over 5,000 calories a day, I had an enormous appetite and snacks were a major part of my life—I couldn't go more than an hour without noshing on something. As a firefighter, snacking helped me pass the hours and soothe the nerves between emergency 911 calls and the frequent amounts of downtime.

However, instead of reaching for the typical range of cookies, donuts, cupcakes, ice cream, candy, and soda pops, which line the countertops and are staples at almost every firehouse, I reach for a variety of healthy snacks that work to enhance my health and my mood rather than hinder them. In fact, snacking on the right foods can keep blood sugar levels stable and prevent gorging at meals. Too many people either don't snack, or forget to snack, and subsequently end up stuffing themselves silly when the pendulum swings the other way.

When the snacks you choose are healthy, you stay healthy and perpetuate a positive cycle of healthy eating.

Here are sixteen of my favorite healthy snack ideas:

1. Fresh fruit: My current favorites are sliced-up watermelon, honeydew, cantaloupe, mangoes, and black grapes. I always have a bowl waiting in the fridge.

2. Vegetables: In my refrigerator you'll almost always find sliced red and green bell peppers, carrots, cucumbers, cherry/cherub tomatoes, and broccoli. I love dipping these in homemade hummus.

3. Whole grain crackers: These days my choice are the Engine 2 Plant-Strong Crispbreads. I often have up to three; the first with a thin layer of no-oil-added peanut butter and low-sugar jam, the second just with jam, and if I have a third, it's naked.

4. Almonds: I'm particularly fond of the Kite Hill brand of fruit-flavored ones. My favorites are strawberry and vanilla.

5. New potatoes: I always make a ton for snacking. These are filling and satiating, especially when dipped in hummus, salsa, or ketchup.

continued

6. Air-popped popcorn with no oil or butter: I've never been a fan of popcorn myself, but I know too many people who go goo-goo over popcorn as a snack, so it's good to have around for healthy guests.

7. Whole grain pretzels: Our shelves at home usually have a box or two.

8. Whole grain Newtons: What a great way to eat a cookie!

9. Chips: Very few on the market have less than 2.5 grams of fat per 100 calories; I like the baked corn tostados from Charras which are super clean. Otherwise, create your own out of pita bread or corn tortillas. Dip them in vitamin-rich salsa.

10. Sliced heirloom tomatoes with balsamic vinegar and cilantro: In the heat of summertime, these refrigerated babies will make you think you've died and gone to heaven.

11. Leftover ears of corn: Sometimes I think these are just as good cold as they are warm—especially in the middle of an Austin summer.

12. Canned fruit: Sometimes I crave a can of mandarin oranges, pears, peaches, or pineapples. However, don't drink the liquid the fruit comes in if it's syrup.

13. Homemade trail mix: 2 cups of Cheerios, ½ cup raw old-fashioned oats, ½ cup chopped dates, ¼ cup raisins, ¼ cup chopped walnuts, ¼ cup chopped almonds: This is a nice concoction to take with you on camping trips, when you're traveling, or when you're just hungry in your own house.

14. Bowl of healthy cereal: I usually munch on a bowl of cereal at some point during the day in addition to my Rip's Big Bowl for breakfast.

15. Salad: I can usually tell when I haven't been eating enough leafy greens because I find myself craving a salad as a snack—I quickly pour an Engine 2 salad dressing over some mixed greens or shredded romaine lettuce along with two or three sliced vegetables.

16. Frozen grapes: These little nuggets of nature make great all-natural popsicles. Pick thirty or forty off the stems and place them in a bowl in the freezer—I can snack on these all day.

E2 DESSERTS

I think it's fair to say most people have a sweet tooth. Myself, I had one coming right out of the gates: My first words weren't "mama" or "dada." They were "more s'mores." No kidding. As I grew older, it didn't matter how much food was in front of me, I always made room for dessert. It was as though I had a second stomach designated for dessert only.

Remember that sugars and sweeteners are full of empty calories. They do have a time and a place in the E2 Diet, however, and that time and place is dessert. If you're anything like me, you need a little something to soothe your sweet tooth (or that second stomach). So here is a smorgasbord of delectable, healthy options to suit your fancy.

E2 Chocolate Knockouts!

Besides tearing into s'mores, when I was growing up I could polish off all the chocolate brownies, chocolate chip cookies, and puddings I could get my little paws on. Even though the following recipes are all healthy, they'll taste as good as your memories of all those other foods that were loaded with nonsense.

E2 Basics Chocolate Mousse

Who doesn't love a great-tasting, healthy chocolate pudding? This is our answer. Scottie suckered our battalion chief (the renowned plant-hater and hard-core meat eater) into having some. He thought it was regular chocolate pudding, never knew the difference, and doesn't to this day!

Serves 2

1 package Mori-Nu silken tofu (lite firm)
2 tablespoons cocoa powder
1 teaspoon vanilla extract
⅓ cup maple syrup

Blend all the ingredients until smooth. Refrigerate until chilled.

Sliced Strawberries and Chocolate Sauce

The flagship Whole Foods Market in Austin resembles an amusement park of food: There are bars for pizza, sushi, Italian food, raw food, salad, sandwiches, smoothies, gelato and ice cream, and the grand finale, a chocolate bar featuring a fountain dripping with luscious chocolate; you can dip anything you want into it.

The chocolate fountain always inspires me to think about mixing chocolate with every possible food, although in my case, it's hard to beat fresh strawberries, which, when I'm not at the store, I dip in this wonderful homemade (dairy-free) chocolate sauce.

Serves 3 to 4 firefighters

1 teaspoon cornstarch
½ cup water
3 tablespoons maple syrup
2 tablespoons cocoa powder
1 teaspoon vanilla extract
2 cups strawberries, sliced

Mix the cornstarch with a small amount of the water in a bowl until there are no lumps. Whisk in the remaining water, syrup, and cocoa. Cook in a heavy saucepan over low heat, stirring continuously until the sauce thickens for 4 to 6 minutes. Remove from the heat and stir in the vanilla. Drizzle the sauce over the strawberries.

Variations:
Stir 1 teaspoon espresso or liqueur into the sauce after removing from heat.
Substitute any fruit for strawberries.

Dark Chocolate Brownies

These brownies are the creation of Engine 2 participant and baker extraordinaire Lydia Heckendorf. Lydia started cooking ten years ago and is a natural at knowing how to make food so terrific tasting no one knows it's healthy as well.

Makes about 20 brownies

1 cup light brown sugar, packed
1 cup unsweetened applesauce
1 tablespoon Ener-G egg replacer mixed with ¼ cup water, or 1 tablespoon ground flaxseed meal mixed with 3 tablespoons warm water
¼ cup plus 2 tablespoons oat or almond milk
1½ teaspoons vanilla extract
1½ teaspoons apple cider vinegar
1½ cups oat flour
1 cup 70 percent (or greater) cocoa powder, unsweetened
1 teaspoon baking soda
½ teaspoon sea salt
1½ cups dairy-free chocolate chips or chunks

Preheat the oven to 375°F. In a large bowl, combine the sugars and applesauce using a fork. Beat in the Ener-G mixture, plant-based milk, vanilla, and vinegar. Combine the dry ingredients (except the chocolate chips) in a separate large bowl. Gradually add the dry mixture to the wet ingredients, then stir in the chocolate chips. Pour the batter into a parchment-lined 9-by-13-inch baking dish. Bake for 16 to 20 minutes and then cool for 5 minutes. These brownies can be gooey so dig in and enjoy!

Simply Chocolate

Here's the easiest dessert of all: Buy any (milk-free) chocolate bar that is 70 percent cocoa or greater. But use restraint! Don't eat the whole bar!

E2 Fresh Fruit and Fruit Bowls

Fresh fruit is a great way to satisfy your sweet tooth and load up on healthy calories filled with antioxidants, fiber, and phytochemicals.

Fruit Bowl with Oat-Nut Topping

Dressing up fruit with some oats and ground nuts adds an interesting and fun twist.

Serves 2

2 bananas, sliced
15-ounce can mandarin orange slices, drained
¼ cup old-fashioned oats
2 tablespoons chopped walnuts

Place the fruit in serving bowls and sprinkle with oats and nuts.

Variation:

Use any favorite sliced fruits to assemble your bowl.

Fruit and Citrus

Slice fresh fruit and place on a small dessert plate. Top with citrus juice or citrus zest and finely chopped mint.

Variations:

Apple slices and lemon juice
Mango slices and lime juice
Kiwi slices and orange juice
Banana slices and grapefruit juice
Blueberries and lemon juice

Fruit Bowl with Soy Drizzle

Add a little plant-based yogurt to fresh or frozen fruit to dress it up for another entertaining twist.

Serves 2

2 bananas, sliced
2 cups fresh or frozen blueberries
4- to 6-ounce container vanilla plant-based yogurt
1 tablespoon maple syrup
½ teaspoon vanilla extract
¼ teaspoon cinnamon

Place the fruit in a bowl. Combine the other ingredients and spoon over the fruit.

Sorbet and Fruit

Simply delicious! Top a scoop of sorbet with fresh or frozen fruit. Use contrasting colors for presentation.

Fruit and Nuts

Enjoy a piece of fruit with 6 to 10 nuts. But remember, nuts are adorable little fat bombs, so use good judgment. And think about getting nuts that are raw and unsalted. Before eating, place them in the toaster oven until browned to bring out the nutty flavor. Just eat a bite of fruit, then a few nuts, and so on.

Variations:
    Nectarines and almonds
    Apples and cashews
    Bananas and walnuts
    Blueberries and pecans

E2 Cobblers, Cookies, and Pies

Scottie is the master baker at Engine 2. He has an uncanny ability to figure out what he wants to make, and poof! It magically appears! Scottie starts by rifling through E2's two refrigerators and twenty-plus food lockers looking for just the right ingredients (in the fire department this common practice is called bird-dogging). Then he pulls out several bowls, spoons, and pans before the tornado strikes. When we ask what he's got in mind, he just tells us to wait and see.

Scottie does it all, from cobblers to cookies, from cakes to pies. Occasionally, when he was in the right mood, he'd let us lend a hand. One time we made dark chocolate chip whole wheat cookies the size of pancakes. We shared several with the A shifters as the shift changed, and two of their wives later asked if they could get the recipe.

Unfortunately, Scottie tends to bake by feel—"using the force" is how he puts it—and so we weren't able to give them the exact recipe. They had to settle for a semblance of one.

Never fear, though, the recipes below are more than a semblance—they are all the real deal.

Blueberry Dumpster Fire Cobbler

My mother loves this recipe because it's so easy to make. The Engine 2 crew calls it Dumpster Fire Cobbler because a Dumpster fire is one of the easiest fires we fight: contained, outdoors, and quickly extinguished with a preconnected booster line on a hose reel. Easy deployment and easy cleanup, just like this cobbler!

Serves 4

$^2/_3$ cup whole wheat pastry flour
1½ teaspoons baking powder
$^2/_3$ cup plant-based milk
3 tablespoons maple syrup
1 tablespoon vanilla extract
2 cups blueberries

Preheat the oven to 350°F. Combine the flour and baking powder in a large bowl. Combine the plant-based milk, syrup, and vanilla in another bowl. Add the wet ingredients to the dry ingredients and mix until smooth. The batter will be runny. Pour the batter into a parchment-lined 8-inch-square pan. Sprinkle the blueberries over the batter. Bake for 45 minutes or until browned.

Variations:
Serve with lemon sorbet.
Substitute any fruit of choice for blueberries.

Fruit Pie with Date-Nut Crust

This fabulous pie was given to us by Austin singer and songwriter Libby Fitzpatrick shortly after our son, Kole, was born. It is sinfully simple and succulently delicious.

Serves 4 to 6

Crust
1 cup dates
⅓ cup walnuts
⅓ cup cashews
⅓ cup almonds
1 teaspoon vanilla extract

Filling
2 or 3 bananas, sliced lengthwise
4 ounces strawberries, sliced
4 ounces strawberries, blended into a puree
4 ounces raspberries
11-ounce can mandarin oranges, drained

Blend the crust ingredients together in a food processor to achieve a sticky consistency. Press the blended crust ingredients into a pie pan. Lay the bananas on top of the crust and press along the sides. Place the strawberry slices on top of the bananas. Pour the strawberry puree over the strawberries and bananas, and press into the gaps. Place the raspberries and mandarin oranges on top of the pie.

Cover and refrigerate for 1 hour or longer before serving.

Chocolate Icebox Pie

This chocolate wonder is so good you may look over your shoulder and see one of Willy Wonka's Oompa Loompas standing on the countertop.

Crust
1 cup dates
1/3 cup walnuts
1/3 cup cashews
1/3 cup almonds
1 teaspoon vanilla extract

Filling
2 bananas, sliced lengthwise
E2 Basics Chocolate Mousse (see page 245)
1 to 2 cups fresh strawberries, sliced, or raspberries

Blend the crust ingredients together in a food processor to achieve a sticky consistency. Press the blended crust ingredients into a pie pan. Lay the bananas on top of the crust and press along the sides. Cover the crust with mousse filling and top with fresh berries to create a healthy chocolate icebox pie! Refrigerate until chilled.

Oatmeal Raisin Cookies

I've always had a special fondness for oatmeal raisin cookies. Another divine creation from Lydia, these will steal the eyes right out of your head.

Makes about 2 dozen

1 cup unsweetened applesauce
2 tablespoons ground flaxseed meal mixed with ¼ cup water
1 cup light brown sugar, packed
1 tablespoon Ener-G egg replacer mixed with ¼ cup water, or 1 table-
    spoon ground flaxseed meal mixed with 3 tablespoons warm water
1 teaspoon vanilla extract
1½ cups whole wheat pastry flour
1 teaspoon ground cinnamon
¼ teaspoon ground nutmeg
1 teaspoon sea salt
1 teaspoon baking soda
3 cups rolled oats
1 cup raisins

Preheat the oven to 375°F. Combine the applesauce, flaxseed mixture, and the sugars with an electric or hand mixer. Beat in the Ener-G mixture and vanilla extract. In a separate large bowl, combine the flour, spices, salt, and baking soda. Gradually mix the wet ingredients into the dry until thoroughly combined. Stir in the oats and raisins. Place rounded, heaping tablespoons of dough onto a parchment-lined cookie sheet and bake for 10 to 12 minutes. Let the cookies cool on a wire rack.

Chocolate Chunk Cookies

If you love chocolate as much as I do, you'll be taken with these.

Makes about 2 dozen

¾ cup plus 2 tablespoons unsweetened applesauce
2 tablespoons ground flaxseed meal mixed with ¼ cup water
1¼ cup light brown sugar, packed
1 tablespoon Ener-G egg replacer mixed with ¼ cup water, or 1 table-
    spoon ground flaxseed meal mixed with 3 tablespoons warm water
1 tablespoon vanilla extract
3 cups whole wheat pastry flour
1 teaspoon baking soda
½ teaspoon sea salt
1½ cups 70 percent cocoa (or greater) dairy-free chocolate chips or chunks

Preheat the oven to 350°F. Mix the applesauce, flaxseed mixture, and sugar together using an electric or hand mixer. Beat in the Ener-G mixture and vanilla. Mix the remaining ingredients (except the chocolate chunks) in a separate large bowl. Gradually add the wet ingredients to the dry ones until thoroughly combined. Stir in the chocolate chunks. Place rounded, heaping tablespoons of dough onto a parchment-lined cookie sheet and bake for 10 to 12 minutes. Let the cookies cool on a wire rack.

E2 Puddings and Mousses

There is something about a really good pudding or mousse that wraps around and clings to every taste bud in your mouth like a generous hug. If you like hugs, you'll like these puddings and mousses.

These are a breeze to whip up and will get you a ton of mileage when it comes to variation in your dessert repertoire.

Fruit Mousse

As mentioned, my childhood pediatrician, Dr. Mercer, finished every checkup by slapping me on the back and saying, "You're healthy as a moose." These fruit mousses are all healthy as a moose, too, and they taste exquisite.

Serves 2

12-ounce package extra-firm Mori-Nu silken tofu
$^1/_3$ cup maple syrup
3 tablespoons fresh fruit juice (see Variations)
Zest of one citrus fruit (see Variations)

Blend all the ingredients together. Cover and refrigerate for an hour or more before serving.

Variations:

Orange Mousse: Use orange juice and zest.

Lime Mousse: Use lime juice and zest.

Mango Mousse: Use 2 fresh mangoes and zest of 1 lime.

Strawberry Mousse: Use 8 ounces fresh or frozen strawberries and zest of 1 orange.

Blueberry Mousse: Use 8 ounces fresh or frozen blueberries, zest of 1 lemon, and 1 teaspoon vanilla.

Maple Sour Cream Dream

The name says it all!

Serves 2

6-ounce vanilla soy or almond yogurt
¼ cup maple syrup
½ teaspoon vanilla extract
8 ounces raspberries

Combine the yogurt, vanilla, and maple syrup. Drizzle over the raspberries.

Variations:

Garnish with raw oats or chopped nuts.
Use blueberries, strawberries, or cherries in place of the raspberries.

Anthony Salerno, 34

Teacher

Coming from an Italian family, I didn't think eating this way was possible for someone with tastes like mine. But I discovered that vegetables without olive oil are better than I ever thought—for the first time, I can really taste them. Best of all, my cholesterol fell from 199 to 140. And I lost nineteen pounds. I never lost that much weight before eating so much, and so happily.

ACKNOWLEDGMENTS

First and foremost, I would like to thank all the fire-fighters from Austin who helped me embark on this wonderful journey over fifteen years ago by teaming up to create delicious and nutritious plant-awesome wagons, including James Rae, Josh Miller, Jeff Dean, Scott Hembree, Scott Walters, Derick Zwerneman, Steve Martinez, Matt Moore, Ali Allazzawi, James Garee, and Craig Walker.

Next, a hearty thank-you to the people in the media who felt that a bunch of firemen eating a plant-powered diet were newsworthy, including Claire Osborn from the *Austin American-Statesman*, the people from National Public Radio, and Deborah Blumenthal from the *New York Times*.

I'd also like to thank the fifty-eight Engine 2 Pilot Study participants who agreed to eat an all-plant-strong diet for six weeks—their dedication to improving their health was impressive, and the results were reflective of their commitment. I am also grateful to the thirteen firefighters and two civilians who participated in the second, twenty-eight-day Pilot Study; I still feel joy from knowing how much their cholesterol levels plummeted and their weight dropped.

I want to thank some very special friends who have been especially supportive: Paul Carrozza from RunTex, for his sage advice, undying optimism, quickness to act, and the name "Engine 2"; Rick Kent, for his constant help with computers, graduation certificates, and photos, and for loving Petey so much; Elizabeth Kreutz, for her photographic expertise; Nathan Turner and John Collis, for exercise expertise; Adam Reiser, for his core workout; Trent Turner, for being medical director for the Pilot Studies; Chad Darbyshire and Josh Miller, for lighting a fire under my butt to do the Pilot Study; the late Seabrook Jones for his enthusiasm; Jared Johnson and Donnie O'Neal, for their creative genius with Engine2.org; Lydia Heckendorf, for her help with the website and the recipe section; Lance Armstrong, for his desire to improve himself in whatever he sinks his teeth into; Anne Stevenson and Tim Terway for being photogenic and brilliant with graphic art design; Brad Kearns, for being a kindred spirit; Bill Stapleton, for coming through and jumping aboard; Dr. Paul Parrish for being so open-minded; Kent Mayes for believing; Charlotte Herzele for her knowledge; Dan, Jackie, and Ryan Murray, for keeping the faith in Windsor, Canada; Darrell Williams for his generosity; the Butler brothers, Adam and Marty, for giving me a place I can call home; Martin Brauns for jumping in feet first; Lyndon Sanders for always putting up a good fight; Ricky Wang for his quiet strength; Jimmy Bynum for being there; the Brinker family for their boldness; Des and Jen Kidd from Port A; and all the guys from Tuesday night choir practice: Rick, John, Adam R., Adam G., Tim, and Chris.

I am so grateful to the crew at Inkwell Management, especially Elisa Petrini and the amazing Richard Pine. Thank you, Richard, for believing in me, taking on the challenge to help make America healthier, and for giving me this wonderful opportunity of a lifetime. Upward and onward! Likewise, I am indebted to all the wonderful folks at Grand Central Publishing, including Jamie Raab, the late Les Pockell, Matthew Ballast, and my superb and supportive editor, Diana Baroni.

Next, a Texas-sized E2 thank-you to Bridget Weiss, for rolling up her sleeves and helping with the proposal, the website, and the recipes. You were there for me 110 percent, and the book wouldn't be the same without you.

I want to thank my brothers, Ted and Zeb; my sister, Jane; my brother-in-law, Brian Hart; my sister-in-law, Anne Bingham; and my two aunts, Susan Lyne and Susan Crile, for their excitement and assistance with anything and everything I've done in life. And of course, my parents, Ann and Essy, for their constant inspiration and love. They are my two greatest role models and I can never get enough of them.

Thank you to the whole Kolasinski clan: Jerry, Carol, John and Basia, and Julie and Pat.

I also want to thank the brave and courageous giants in this field who have paved the way and given me the courage to stand up and be heard: my father, T. Colin Campbell, Dean Ornish, Neal Barnard, John McDougall, Joel Fuhrman, and Jeff Novick.

Without my wife and love, Jill Kolasinski, I don't know how I could have managed this project. Thank you, Jill, for your unwavering love and support. And huge hugs and kisses to my son, Kole, and my daughters, Sophie and Hope, for stampeding into our lives and teaching us how to live life to the plant-strong max!

Finally, I want to thank my co-writer, advisor, and friend, Gene Stone. In your brilliant little ways you knew how to bring out the best in me. You are indeed a holy ghost. Boy, did we have fun creating this baby! I will always treasure the time we spent working on the book, and the professional and personal relationship we were able to forge.

INDEX

abdominal fat, 104–5
added fats, on food labels, 116–17
added sodium, on food labels, 114
added sugars, on food labels, 114–15
alcohol, 30, 67
Alfredo Sauce, Linguine and Creamy, 195
Almighty Healthy Wrap, 171–72
almond milk, 24, 30, 132
almonds, 124, 243
    dessert recipes, 251–52
Alzheimer's disease, 62–65
    plant-based diet and research, 63–65
    risk factors for, 64–65
    statistics on, 62–63
American diet and diseases, xi, 7, 11, 13, 14, 22, 42–43. *See also specific diseases*
American-Style Plant-Strong Brats, 166–67
angina, 45, 47
Ann's Panini with Hummus, Mushrooms, and Spinach, 165
antioxidants, 55, 67
Arm Circles, 75
Armstrong, Lance, 16, 95
Asian Marinade, 241
Asparagus, Cravotta's Couscous with Tomatoes and, 183–84
athletic performance, 9–10
    and plant-based diet myth, 36–37
attitude, 89–95, 126

avocados. *See also* guacamole
    in Basics Salad, 173
    in Black Beans and Rice, 178
    in Mexican Lime Soup, 218–19
    preparation tip, 139–40
    in Rip's Sweet Potato Bowl, 227
    storage tips, 142

Baby Field Greens Salad, 172–73
Barnard, Neal, 58–59, 92
Barrel Rolls, 75
Basics Chocolate Mousse, 245
Basics Dressing, 232
Basics Open-Faced Sandwich, 164
Basics Pancakes, 158
Basics Pita, 168–69
Basics Salad, 173
Basics Tacos, 223
Basics Wrap, 169
BBQ Pizza, Bert's, 200–201
Beam Me Up, Scottie, Dressing, 234
beans (legumes), 32, 67. *See also specific types of beans*
    cooking tips, 138–39
    in Plant-Strong Brats, 166–67
    recommended canned, 131
    Three-Bean Chili, 220–21
beef. *See* meat
Bert's BBQ Pizza, 200–201
beta-amyloid, 63
beta-carotene, 50, 64, 190
big salads, recipes, 212–16

black beans
in Almighty Healthy Wrap, 171–72
in Basics Tacos, 223
Black Beans and Rice, 177–78
Black Bean Spread, 235
in Breakfast Tacos, 155
in EMS Portobello Mushroom Fajitas
with Rice and Guacamole, 228
in Great Wooden Bowl Salad, 214–15
in Jane's Jammin' Burritos, 229
in Nachos, 226
in New York Times Veggie Burgers, 186
in Picadillo Pick Ax Burrito, 224
in Rip's Sweet Potato Bowl, 227
blood pressure, 102–3
high. *See* hypertension
ideal goal, 102
stroke risk and, 49–50
blood testing, 94–95
Blueberry Dumpster Fire Cobbler, 250–51
Blueberry Mousse, 255
Blueberry Spelt Pancakes, 159
body fat, 21, 54
percentage body fat, 104–5
body mass index (BMI), 103–4
books, recommended, 92
bowel movements, 20–21, 55, 67
Bow Ties with Pesto, 196
Bran Muffins, Quick, 161
bran of whole grain, 118
Brats, Plant-Strong, 166–67
breads, 34–35
anatomy of, 118
recommended brands, 129–30, 131
breakfast, importance of, 149–50
breakfast recipes, 149–62
fruit and toast, 162
hearty cereal bowls, 150–52
Saturday specials, 152–57
Sunday morning pancakes and muffins,
157–61
Breakfast Tacos, 155

breast cancer, 52, 54, 138
Brinker, Jeff, 98
broccoli, 36, 67
in Green Pizza, 197–98
in Pad Thai, 211
in Raise-the-Roof Sweet Potato-
Vegetable Lasagna, 202–3
Brooks, Aaron, 93
broths, 134, 138
Brownies, Dark Chocolate, 247
brown rice, 142
cooking methods, 175–77
Black Beans and Rice, 177–78
Candle Café Brown Rice and Lentil
Burgers, 188–89
EMS Portobello Mushroom Fajitas with
Rice and Guacamole, 228
in Jane's Jammin' Burritos, 229
in Plant-Strong Brats, 166–67
recommended brands, 129, 133–34
Red Vegetable Curry and Brown Rice,
210–11
in Rice Salad, 212
in Rip's Big Leaf Special, 170
Vegetable Stir-Fry with Brown Rice, 208
Brussels sprouts, 67
in Rip's Roasted Salad, 216
Burbies, 79
burgers
Candle Café Brown Rice and Lentil
Burgers, 188–89
EZ Burgers, 184–85
New York Times Veggie Burgers, 186
Portobello Mushroom Burgers, 187
burger substitutes, 28, 184
burritos
Basics Burrito, 223
Jane's Jammin' Burritos, 229
Picadillo Pick Ax Burrito, 224
recommended brands, 133
butter, 24, 103, 135, 141
Butz, John, 5–6

calcium, 26, 32
calories, overview, 61–62
Campbell, T. Colin, xi–xiii, 36–37, 47–48, 52, 55, 92
cancer, 51–55, 138
    causes of, 51–52
    diet promoting, 52–53
    plant-based diet and research, 52, 54–55
Candle Café Brown Rice and Lentil Burgers, 188–89
candles, as fire risk, 66
Cannellini Dip, 237
caramelizing onions, 137
carbohydrates
    calories in, 61–62
    myth about fat and, 34–35
cardiovascular disease. *See* heart disease; strokes
cardiovascular exercises, 70, 76, 79, 82, 85–86, 98
Carl Sandburg stretches, 72–75, 86
Carmona, Richard, 60
casein, 24, 52, 135
cashews
    in Linguine and Creamy Alfredo Sauce, 195
    in Mac-N-Cash, 207
    Roasted Bell Peppers, Baked Sweet Potatoes, and Galloping Greens with Cashew Sauce, 181–82
casomorphines, 24
Castelli, William, 48
cauliflower
    Kole's Creamy Cauliflower Soup, 219–20
    in Rip's Roasted Salad, 216
cereal bowls, recipes, 150–52
cereals, recommended brands, 127–29, 131–32
Chalupas, 225
cheese, 24–25, 103, 135
cheese substitutes, 24, 135

chickpeas
    in Healthy Homemade Hummus, 236
    in Spinach Salad with Healthy Homemade Croutons, 213–14
    Three-Bean Chili, 220–21
children, and plant-based diet myth, 38
chiles, roasting, 139
Chili, Three-Bean, 220–21
China Study, The (Campbell), 36–37, 47–48, 52, 92
Chinese cuisine, 125
chips, 28, 244
Chocolate Chunk Cookies, 254
chocolate desserts, recipes, 245–47
Chocolate Icebox Pie, 252
Chocolate Mousse, Basics, 245
cholesterol, 12, 25, 100. *See also* HDL cholesterol; LDL cholesterol
    Alzheimer's risk and, 64
    Engine 2 Pilot Studies, 18, 19, 20, 27
    heart disease risk and, 48
    hypertension risk and, 103
    ideal goal, 13, 48, 100
    JR's results, 15–17
Cleveland Clinic, 11–12, 13
Cobbler, Blueberry Dumpster Fire, 250–51
collard greens, 67, 140, 170–71
comfort dinners, recipes, 201–7
complex carbohydrates, 34–35
condiments, 132, 235
constipation, 18, 42
Continental Marinade, 242
cookies
    Chocolate Chunk Cookies, 254
    Oatmeal Raisin Cookies, 253
    substitutes, 28
cooking sprays, 24, 110, 138
cooking tips, 136–40
core exercises, 78, 81–82, 84–85

corn, 32
  in Almighty Healthy Wrap, 171–72
  in Mexican Lime Soup, 218–19
  in Picadillo Pick Ax Burrito, 224
  in Rice Salad, 212
corn syrups, 115, 135
coronary blockages, 45, 46, 47
Couscous with Tomatoes and Asparagus,
    Cravotta's, 183–84
crackers, 67, 95, 111, 243
Cravotta, Audrey, 71
Cravotta, Mark, 183, 219
Cravotta, Monica, 185, 219
Cravotta's Couscous with Tomatoes and
    Asparagus, 183–84
Creamy Green Avocado Dressing, 234
Crile, George, Sr., 11, 13
Crile, George "Barney," Jr., 13,
    50–51, 72
Crow, Joseph, 12–13
Curry and Brown Rice, Red Vegetable,
    210–11

dairy, 24–25, 28–29, 135
  calcium myth, 35
  cancer risk and, 52
  diabetes risk and, 56
  fat content, on packages, 108–9
dairy substitutes, 24, 28–29, 134, 141
dark chocolate, 25, 28, 30, 247
Dark Chocolate Brownies, 247
Davis, LD, 43–44
Dellert, Alphonse, "Ax," 4–6
DeMan, Renee, 166
dementia, 62–65
  plant-based diet and research, 63–65
desserts, 30, 125
dessert recipes, 245–56
  chocolate, 245–47
  cobblers, cookies, and pies, 250–54
  fruit, 248–49
  puddings and mousses, 255–56

diabetes, 55–59
  fasting glucose/blood sugar, 102
  plant-based diet and research, 58–59
  statistics on, 55–56
Dijon Dressing, 232
dinner recipes, 175–231
  big salads, 212–16
  burgers, 184–89
  comfort foods, 201–7
  dinner plates, 177–84
  pasta, 192–96
  pizza, 196–201
  potato sides, 190–91
  soups, 217–22
  stir-fries, 208–11
  Tex-Mex, 222–31
dips, recipes, 235–41
disease prevention, 67
Downward Dogs, 83–84
dressings, recipes, 232–34

E2 Almighty Healthy Wrap, 171–72
E2 attitude, 89–95, 126
E2 Basics Chocolate Mousse, 245
E2 Basics Dressing, 232
E2 Basics Pancakes, 158
E2 Basics Pita, 168–69
E2 Basics Salad, 173
E2 Basics Tacos, 223
E2 Basics Wrap, 169
E2 Black Beans and Rice,
    177–78
E2 Brown Rice, 175–77
E2 Easy Weekly Planner, 143–45
E2 EZ Burgers, 184–85
E2 Hot Lap Bowl, 151
E2 Omelet, 156–57
E2 Sour Cream, 239
eating out, 123–26
Eat to Live (Fuhrman), 32, 92
eggs, 26, 53
Elkind, Mitchell, 50

EMS Portobello Mushroom Fajitas with
  Rice and Guacamole, 228
Enchiladas, Matt Moore's, 230–31
endosperm of whole grain, 118
energy levels, 25
  plant-based diet myth about, 37–38
Engine 2 Diet
  benefits of, 15, 21–22, 27
  Fire Cadet plan, 22–23
  Firefighter plan, 22, 23–29
  medical proof behind, 41–67
  mission statement, 119–20
  myths about, 31–40
  overview of, 21
Engine 2 Exercise Program. *See* exercise
  program
Engine 2 Firehouse, 15–16, 57, 60, 69–70,
  94, 163, 171, 188–89, 190, 194, 196,
  200, 228, 230, 240
  Lake Shore Apartments fire, 3–7
Engine 2 Pilot Studies, 11, 17–21, 27,
  39, 99
erectile dysfunction, 39
escape plan, in case of fire, 66
Esselstyn, Ann, 13, 165, 167, 197, 250
Esselstyn, Caldwell B., Jr., xii, xiii, 9–10,
  11–13, 39, 46, 99
Esselstyn, Caldwell B., Sr., 11
Esselstyn, Jane, 201, 229, 237
Esselstyn, Kole, 204, 219, 251
Esselstyn, Ted and Zeb, 201
essential amino acids, 33–34, 62, 64
exercise, benefits of, 67, 70
exercise program, 69–86, 98
  before getting started, 72
  round 1, 77–80
  round 2, 80–82
  round 3, 82–86
  scheduling chart, 76
  warm down, 86
  warm up, 72–75
EZ Burgers, 184–85

Fajitas with Rice and Guacamole, EMS
  Portobello Mushroom, 228
fasting glucose/blood sugar, 102
fat(s)
  calories in, 61–62
  plant-based diet myth about, 36
fat claims, on food packages, 108–12
fat content, on food labels, 113, 116–17
"fat free," on food packages, 110
fiber, 22, 55, 67, 140
  carbohydrates and, 34–35
  on food labels, 117–18
Fire Cadet plan, 22–23
fire extinguishers, 66
Firefighter plan, 22, 23–29
  week one, 24–25
  week three, 26–27
  week two, 25–26
fire prevention, 66–67
fish, 25, 28, 180
fish oil supplements, 38–39
Fitzpatrick, Libby, 251
flaxseed meal, 142
Flutter Kicks, 78
food cravings, 93
food labels. *See* label reading
food logs, 99
food myths, 31–40
food substitutes, 140–41
food taste, 20, 27, 39–40
forgiving yourself, 93
free radicals, 38, 53, 55
French Toast, 153
Fresh Fruit Extravaganza with Mint, 162
friends, support from, 90, 92
Frost, Cindy, 93
fruits. *See also specific fruits*
  as healthy snacks, 243, 244
  recipes, 248–49
  storage tips, 142
  time-saver tips, 142
Fruit and Citrus, 248

Fruit and Nuts, 249
Fruit and Sorbet, 249
Fruit Bowl with Oat-Nut
    Topping, 248
Fruit Bowl with Soy Drizzle, 249
Fruit Extravaganza with Mint,
    Fresh, 162
Fruit Mousse, 255
Fruit Pie with Date-Nut Crust, 251–52
Fuhrman, Joel, 32, 92
Funky Feet Jumping Jacks, 82

gallstones, 43
Garee, James, 36, 51
germ of whole grain, 118
Gill, Kin, 54
Gingered Mushrooms, Bok Choy, and
    Carrots with Soba Noodles, 205
glucose, 34–35, 56–58
    fasting glucose/blood sugar, 102
Gnocchi and Red Sauce, 192
Gonzalez, Tony, 36–37
grain type, on food packages, 111
grapes, frozen, for snacking, 244
Great Wooden Bowl Salad, 214–15
Greek Pizza, 199
green leafy vegetables, 27, 35, 39, 50, 67.
    See also specific greens
    preparation tip, 140
    storage tips, 141–42
Green Leafy Wrap, 170–71
Green Pizza, 197–98
grilling vegetables, 137–38
guacamole, 28
    EMS Portobello Mushroom Fajitas with
        Rice and Guacamole, 228
    in Nachos, 226
    recipe, 238–39

hash brown potatoes, frozen
    in Breakfast Tacos, 155
    in Matt Moore's Enchiladas, 230–31

HDL cholesterol, 100–101
    Engine 2 Pilot Studies, 18, 19, 20, 27
    ideal goal, 100–101
headaches, 42
Healthy Homemade Hummus, 236
"healthy," on food packages, 111–12
heart disease, 43–49
    causes of, 45–46
    cholesterol levels and, 17
    diabetes and, 56
    Esselstyn, Jr.'s research, xii,
        11–12, 46
    LD's story, 43–44
    plant-based diet and research, 46–49
heart rate step test, 3-minute, 105–6
hearty cereal bowls, recipes, 150–52
Heckendorf, Lydia, 247, 253
Heidrich, Ruth, 37
hemorrhagic strokes, 38, 49
high blood pressure. *See* hypertension
homocysteine, 64
Hot Lap Bowl, 151
hummus, 28, 132
    in Almighty Healthy Wrap, 171–72
    Ann's Panini with Hummus,
        Mushrooms, and Spinach, 165
    in Basics Wrap, 169
    in Green Leafy Wrap, 170–71
    Healthy Homemade Hummus, 236
    in Kale, Lemon, and Cilantro Sandwich,
        167–68
    in Rip's Big Leaf Special, 170
hydrogenated oils, 111, 116–17
hypertension, 102–3
    Alzheimer's risk and, 64
    heart disease risk and, 48

Icebox Pie, Chocolate, 252
impotence, 39
insulin, 21, 25, 34–35, 56–57, 59
insulin-like growth factor-1 (IGF-1), 52
ischemic strokes, 49

Island Marinade, 241
Italian cuisine, 125. *See also* pasta

jackfruit, 26, 28
Jane's Jammin' Burritos, 229
Japanese cuisine, 125
Jocelyn, Carol, 59
Jocelyn, Lynn, 204
Jumping Jacks, 82

kale, 67
    Kale, Lemon, and Cilantro Sandwich,
      167–68
    Kale Butter, 237
    in Pasta Primavera, 194
    Red Beans over Quinoa with Kale, 178–79
key nutrients, and plant-based diet myth, 37
Kicking Toe Touches, 73
kitchen
    cooking tips, 136–40
    foods to remove, 134–35
    pantry ingredients, 127–34
    Whole Foods Brand Foods, 131–34
kitchen tools, 135–36
Kolasinski, Jill, 38, 90, 137, 178, 202, 204,
    214, 219
Kole's Creamy Cauliflower Soup, 219–20
Kuller, Lewis, 45

label reading, 107–18
    "nutritional facts" label, 108, 112–18
    typical claims made on outside of
      package, 108–12
lactose intolerance, 25
LaFuente, Tim, 202
LaLanne, Jack, 31
Lasagna, Raise-the-Roof Sweet Potato-
    Vegetable, 202–3
LDL cholesterol, 100–101
    Engine 2 Pilot Studies, 18, 19, 20, 27
    ideal goal, 13, 48, 100–101
leg exercises, 77, 80, 82–83

legumes. *See* beans
lemons, 125
    Kale, Lemon, and Cilantro Sandwich,
      167–68
    Lemon Cornmeal Pancakes, 157
    protein value, 201
lentils
    Candle Café Brown Rice and Lentil
      Burgers, 188–89
    cooking tip, 139
    Lynn's Meatloaf, 204
    Savory Lentils and Greens, 222
    in Shepherd's Pie, 206–7
    in Sloppy Joes, 188
Liebowitz, Linda, 65
Liebowitz, Matthew, 25
Lime Mousse, 255
Lime Soup, Mexican, 218–19
Linguine and Creamy Alfredo Sauce, 195
lunch recipes, 163–75
    salads, 172–75
    sandwiches, 163–68
    wraps and pitas, 168–77
Lunges, 80
Lynn's Meatloaf, 204

McDougall, John, xii–xiii, 35, 52, 54, 62, 92
Mac-N-Cash, 207
mangoes
    Mango Mousse, 255
    preparation tip, 139
    in Red Tip Lettuce Salad, 174
    in Rip's Sweet Potato Bowl, 227
Maple Sour Cream Dream, 256
marinades, recipes, 241–42
Marsh, Brandon and Amy, 40
Martinez, Steve, 22, 51, 188, 210, 220
Matt Moore's Enchiladas, 230–31
mayonnaise, 28, 235
meal planner, 143–45
meat, 25, 28, 32–33, 53, 94, 135
Meatloaf, Lynn's, 204

meat substitutes, 26, 140–41
medical proof, 41–67
  Alzheimer's disease/dementia, 62–65
  cancer, 51–55
  diabetes, 55–59
  heart disease, 43–49
  obesity, 60–62
  stroke, 49–51
methionine, 64
Mexican cuisine, 125
  Tex-Mex favorites, recipes, 154, 222–31
Mexican Lime Soup, 218–19
Mexican Marinade, 242
Mexican-Style Plant-Strong Brats, 166–67
Migas Especiales, 154
Mighty Muffins, 160
milk, 24–25, 28–29, 135
  cancer risk and, 52
  diabetes risk and, 56
  fat content, on packages, 108–9
milk substitutes, 24, 62, 141
Miller, Josh, 4, 6, 15, 16, 22, 112
mirin, 136–37, 205
mission statement, 119–20
monounsaturated fats, 26–27
Moore, Matt, 158, 210, 220, 230
Moses, Edwin, 10
Moskowitz, Isa Chandra, 157
motivation, 91
Mountain Climbers, 85–86
mousses, recipes, 245, 255–56
muffins
  Mighty Muffins, 160
  Quick Bran Muffins, 161
muscular system, and exercise, 70–71
mushrooms, 32
  in Almighty Healthy Wrap, 171–72
  Ann's Panini with Hummus,
    Mushrooms, and Spinach, 165
  in E2 Omelet, 156–57
  EMS Portobello Mushroom Fajitas with
    Rice and Guacamole, 228

Gingered Mushrooms, Bok Choy, and
    Carrots with Soba Noodles, 205
  grilling, 138
  in Matt Moore's Enchiladas, 230–31
  in Mexican Lime Soup, 218–19
  Mushroom Stroganoff, 193
  Portobello Mushroom Burgers, 187
  Tempeh-Mushroom Stir-Fry and Soba
    Noodles, 209
  Tofu Steaks and Mushrooms with
    Mashed Potatoes and Green Beans,
    180–81
myths about food, 31–40

Nachos, 226
"natural," on food packages, 111–12
Navratilova, Martina, 10, 37
New York Times Veggie Burgers, 186
nitroglycerin pills, 45
"nonfat," on food packages, 110
nonstick sprays, 24, 110, 138
Novick, Jeff, 107
nuts, 35, 142. See also specific nuts
  Fruit and Nuts, 249
  storage tips, 142
  toasting, 139
nut butters, 142
"nutritional facts" label, 108, 112–18
nutritional yeast, 28, 198

oatmeal
  Oatmeal Raisin Cookies, 253
  protein value, 32
  Quick Oatmeal Bowl, 152
  recommended brands, 129, 132
obesity, xi, 60–62
  Alzheimer's risk and, 64
  carbohydrates and fat myth, 34–35
  heart disease risk and, 48
  plant-based diet and research, 61–62
  statistics on, 60
oils, 26–27, 29, 53, 135

olive oil, 26–27, 39
omega-3 fatty acids, 25, 38–39
Omelet, E2, 156–57
onions, caramelizing, 137
Orange Hummus Dressing, 234
Orange Mousse, 255
Ornish, Dean, 32, 46–47, 54
osteoporosis, 35, 42, 71
ovarian cancer, 52, 53, 242
oxidants, 46, 53

Pad Thai, 211
palate, 20, 27, 39–40
pancakes
    E2 Basics Pancakes, 158
    Lemon Cornmeal Pancakes, 157
    Spelt Blueberry Pancakes, 159
Panini with Hummus, Mushrooms, and
    Spinach, Ann's, 165
pantry foods to remove, 134–35
pantry ingredients, recommended brands,
    127–34
partners, support from, 90, 92
pasta, 192–96
    Bow Ties with Pesto, 196
    Gnocchi and Red Sauce, 192
    Linguine and Creamy Alfredo Sauce, 195
    Mac-N-Cash, 207
    Mushroom Stroganoff, 193
    Pasta Primavera, 194
    Raise-the-Roof Sweet Potato-Vegetable
        Lasagna, 202–3
    recommended brands, 129,
        133–34
Pasta Primavera, 194
PB and Banana, 162
Peanut Dressing, 233
percentage body fat, 104–5
pesto
    Bow Ties with Pesto, 196
    in Greek Pizza, 199
phytochemicals, 46, 55, 67

Picadillo Pick Ax Burrito, 224
pies, recipes, 251–52
Pike-Ups, 84–85
pitas, 168–77
    Basics Pita, 168–69
pizza, 196–201
    Bert's BBQ Pizza, 200–201
    Greek Pizza, 199
    eating out, 125
    Green Pizza, 197–98
    substitutes, 28
    Supreme Pizza, 197
pizza crusts, recommended brands,
        129–30, 131
Plank Pose, 81–82
plant-based diet. *See also* Engine 2 Diet
    author's story, 9–11
    author's studies, 11, 17–21, 41
    benefits of, xi–xiii, 21–22
    Esselstyn, Jr.'s research, xii, 11–12, 39
    myths about, 31–40
Plant-Strong Brats, 166–67
plaque formations, 45, 46, 47, 63
Pondo, Marisa, 28
popcorn, 244
Portobello Mushroom Burgers, 187
Portobello Mushroom Fajitas with Rice
        and Guacamole, 228
positive attitude, 89–95, 126
potassium, 50
potatoes, 32. *See also* sweet potatoes
    in Kole's Creamy Cauliflower Soup,
        219–20
    Potato Wedges, 190–91
    in Rip's Roasted Salad, 216
    in Shepherd's Pie, 206–7
    Steamed Red Potatoes, 191
    Tofu Steaks and Mushrooms with
        Mashed Potatoes and Green Beans,
        180–81
Potato Wedges, 190–91
pretzels, 124, 244

pregnant mothers, and plant-based diet
myth, 38
Prevent and Reverse Heart Disease
(Esselstyn. Jr.), 12, 92
prostate cancer, 52, 54, 138
protein, 9, 32–34
calories in, 61–62
harm of animal-based, 32
plant-based diet myths about, 32–34
recommended, 32
PSA (prostate-specific antigen), 54
puddings, recipes, 255–56
Push-Ups, 77–78

Quick Bran Muffins, 161
Quick Oatmeal Bowl, 152
quinoa, 129, 142
Red Beans over Quinoa with Kale,
178–79

Rae, James "JR," 15–17, 112
Raise-the-Roof Sweet Potato-Vegetable
Lasagna, 202–3
Ray, Rachael, 193
real men, and plant-based diet myth, 39
recipes, 149–256. *See also*
specific recipes
breakfasts, 149–62
desserts, 245–56
dinner, 175–231
dressings spreads, and marinades,
232–42
lunches, 163–75
time-saver tips, 142
Red Beans over Quinoa with Kale,
178–79
red meat. *See* meat
Red Tip Lettuce Salad, 174
Red Vegetable Curry and Brown Rice,
210–11
refined sugars, 114–15, 135
reframing the picture, 92–93

refried beans
in Chalupas, 225
in Jane's Jammin' Burritos, 229
in Migas Especiales, 154
resistance/strength training, 70–71
restaurants, 123–26
rice. *See* brown rice
Rice Salad, 212
Rip's Big Bowl, 150–51
Rip's Big Leaf Special, 170
Rip's Roasted Salad, 216
Rip's Sweet Potato Bowl, 227
RMR (resting metabolic rate), 71, 98
Roasted Bell Peppers, Baked Sweet
Potatoes, and Galloping Greens with
Cashew Sauce, 181–82
Roasted Salad, Rip's, 216
roasting peppers and fresh chilies, 139

salads, 172–75, 212–16, 244
Baby Field Greens Salad, 172–73
E2 Basics Salad, 173
Great Wooden Bowl Salad, 214–15
Red Tip Lettuce Salad, 174
Rice Salad, 212
Rip's Roasted Salad, 216
Spinach Salad, 175
Spinach Salad with Healthy Homemade
Croutons, 213–14
Spring Greens Salad, 174
salad dressings, recipes, 232–34
Salerno, Anthony, 39, 159, 256
salsa, 28, 125, 134
in Breakfast Tacos, 155
in Migas Especiales, 154
recipe, 240
Southwest Salsa, 240–41
salt. *See* sodium
salt substitutes, 141
Sampson, McClain, 98, 100
Sanchez, Celia, 242
Sanchez, Jessica, 242

Sandburg stretches, 72–75, 86
sandwiches, 163–68
  Ann's Panini with Hummus,
    Mushrooms, and Spinach, 165
  Basics Open-Faced Sandwich, 164
  Kale, Lemon, and Cilantro Sandwich,
    167–68
  Plant-Strong Brats, 166–67
  Sloppy Joes, 188
saturated fats, 26–27, 52, 61–62, 64, 103
sautéing tip, 137
Savory Lentils and Greens, 222
Scott, Dave, 9–10, 37, 91
Seated Chair Dips, 80–81
Seated V-Ups, 84–85
seitan, 26, 28, 141
  in Vegetable Stir-Fry with Brown
    Rice, 208
self-motivation, 91
"servings per container," on food labels,
  112–13
Sesame Seed Dressing, 233
sexual dysfunction, 39
Shepherd's Pie, 206–7
Side Stretches, 74
Simple Cereal Bowl, 152
Sliced Strawberries and Chocolate
  Sauce, 246
Sloppy Joes, 188
smoke detectors, 66
smoking, 31, 48, 67
snacks, 67, 95, 124, 243
  healthy ideas, 243–44
soba noodles
  Gingered Mushrooms, Bok Choy, and
    Carrots with Soba Noodles, 205
  Tempeh-Mushroom Stir-Fry and Soba
    Noodles, 209
soda, 28, 29, 113, 115, 125, 135
sodium (salt), 50, 103
  on food labels, 114
  substitutes, 141

sorbet, 28, 125
Sorbet and Fruit, 249
soups, 134, 217–22
  Kole's Creamy Cauliflower Soup,
    219–20
  Mexican Lime Soup, 218–19
  Savory Lentils and Greens, 222
  Split Pea Soup, 217
Sour Cream, 239
Southwest Salsa, 240–41
soybeans, 36, 39, 140, 209
soy cheese, 24
Spelt Blueberry Pancakes, 159
spices, 141, 142
spinach, 32, 36
  in Almighty Healthy Wrap, 171–72
  Ann's Panini with Hummus,
    Mushrooms, and Spinach, 165
  in Bert's BBQ Pizza, 200–201
  in E2 Omelet, 156
  in Green Pizza, 197–98
  in Matt Moore's Enchiladas, 230–31
  Spinach Salad, 175
  Spinach Salad with Healthy Homemade
    Croutons, 213–14
Split Pea Soup, 217
Spock, Benjamin, 38
spreads, recipes, 235–41
Spring Greens Salad, 174
Squat Thrusts, 79
Steamed Red Potatoes, 191
steaming tip, 137
Step-Ups, 82–83
stir-fries, recipes, 208–11
  Pad Thai, 211
  Red Vegetable Curry and Brown Rice,
    210–11
  Tempeh-Mushroom Stir-Fry and Soba
    Noodles, 209
  Vegetable Stir-Fry with Brown Rice,
    208
stir-frying, about, 136–37, 208

storage tips, 141–42
Stoudamire, Salim, 37
strawberries, 36
  in Fruit Pie with Date-Nut Crust,
    251–52
  Sliced Strawberries and Chocolate
    Sauce, 246
  Strawberry Mousse, 255
strength/resistance training, 70–71
strengths, playing to your, 93–94
stretching exercises, 72–75, 86
Stroganoff, Mushroom, 193
strokes, 49–51
  causes of, 49–50
  diabetes and, 56
  plant-based diet and research,
    50–51
  statistics on, 49
Sun Salutations, 73, 86
support groups, 92
Supreme Pizza, 197
sweeteners, 141
sweet potatoes
  Raise-the-Roof Sweet Potato-Vegetable
    Lasagna, 202–3
  Rip's Sweet Potato Bowl, 227
  Roasted Bell Peppers, Baked Sweet
    Potatoes, and Galloping Greens with
    Cashew Sauce, 181–82
  Sweet Potato Fries, 190–91
  Sweet Potato Rounds, 191

tacos
  Basics Tacos, 223
  Breakfast Tacos, 155
tempeh, 28, 141
  Tempeh-Mushroom Stir-Fry and Soba
    Noodles, 209
Tex-Mex favorites, recipes, 154,
  222–31
Thai cuisine, 125
  Pad Thai, 211

3-minute heart rate step test, 105–6
Three-Bean Chili, 220–21
TIAs (transient ischemic attacks), 49, 63
time-saver tips, 142
Tinley, Scott, 91
toasting nuts and seeds, 139
toasts, recipes, 153, 162
tofu, 26, 28, 140–41
  in Basics Chocolate Mousse, 245
  in E2 Omelet, 156–57
  in Fruit Mousse, 255
  in Great Wooden Bowl Salad,
    214–15
  in Migas Especiales, 154
  in Red Vegetable Curry and Brown Rice,
    210–11
  in Sour Cream, 239
  Tofu Steaks and Mushrooms with
    Mashed Potatoes and Green Beans,
    180–81
  Tofu Vegetable Spread, 238
tortillas
  recommended brands, 129–30, 131
  warming up, 139
trail mix, 244
trans fats, 111, 116–17
traveling and eating out, 124–26
treadmill stress test, 20
triglycerides, 101
  Engine 2 Pilot Studies, 18, 19, 20
  ideal goal, 101
Trunk Twists, 74
"2 percent (or 1 percent) fat," on food
    packages, 108–9
type 1 diabetes, 56
type 2 diabetes, 57–59, 102

Vasquez, Arty, 92
vegetables. *See also specific vegetables*
  cooking tips, 136–38
  cutting, slicing, and chopping, 136
  for snacking, 243

storage tips, 141–42
time-saver tips, 142
Vegetable Stir-Fry with Brown Rice, 208
Vegetable Stock, Homemade, 138
vegetarian diet. *See* Engine 2 Diet;
    plant-based diet
Veggie Burgers, New York Times, 186
vices and virtues, 30
vital signs, 18, 97–106
    blood pressure, 102–3
    body mass index, 103–4
    fasting glucose/blood sugar, 102
    food logs, 99
    LDL and HDL cholesterol, 100–101
    percentage body fat, 104–5
    3-minute heart rate step test, 105–6
    total cholesterol, 100
    triglycerides, 101
    weight, 97–98
vitamin B2, 50
vitamin B12, 37, 62, 198
vitamin C, 50
vitamin E, 50
V-Ups, 84–85

Walker, Craig, 59, 92, 93–94
Wallis, Colin J., 21
walnuts
    in Bow Ties with Pesto, 196
    in Fruit Bowl with Oat-Nut Topping, 248

in Kale Butter, 237
in Spinach Salad with Healthy
    Homemade Croutons, 213–14
Walters, Scott "Scottie," 51, 210, 230, 234,
    245, 250
warm down, 86
warm ups, 72–75
Weekly Planner, 143–45
weight checks, 97–98
weight gain, 61. *See also* obesity
weight lifting, 31, 70–71
weight loss, xi, 97–98
    benefit of Engine 2 Diet, 21
    Engine 2 Pilot Studies, 18, 19, 20
wheat gluten. *See* seitan
whole grains, 26, 34, 67
    anatomy of, 118
    claims on food packages, 111
    recommended brands, 129–30, 133–34
wraps, 168–77
    E2 Almighty Healthy Wrap, 171–72
    E2 Basics Wrap, 169
    Green Leafy Wrap, 170–71
    Rip's Big Leaf Special, 170
    warming up, 139

"zero trans fat," on food packages,
    110–11
Zwerneman, Derick, 22, 152–53, 163, 181,
    188, 210, 220